Thirty Essential Tips To Start Managing The Alzheimer's Or Other Dementia, Your Parent, and Yourself

Thirty Essential Tips To Start Managing The Alzheimer's Or Other Dementia, Your Parent, and Yourself

AN ELDER CARE SURVIVAL GUIDE

Charlotte Keys

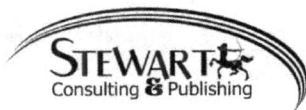

STEWART
Consulting & Publishing

Available from Amazon.com, Createspace.com, and Stewartpublishing.com

Thirty Essential Tips to Start Managing the Alzheimer's or Other Dementia, Your Parent, and Yourself:
An Elder Care Survival Guide

© 2017 by Charlotte Keys

Disclaimer: The information in this book is presented solely for educational purposes. It is not intended to serve as medical or legal advice or to replace the advice and counsel of a doctor and attorney. Neither the publisher nor the author is responsible for any adverse consequences resulting from the use of any of the suggestions discussed in this book.

Library of Congress Control Number: 2017902600

Stewart Consulting & Publishing Inc., Hazel Crest, IL

ISBN-10: 069284984X

ISBN-13: 9780692849842

Dedication

In memory of my mom and dad

and

For all of us, their kids and grandkids, still strewn about the country, still missing them

Acknowledgements

First, I would like to thank the hard-working members of the organizations that follow. They have shown great dedication to making medical and healthcare information available and easily accessible to the general public. Their published websites have both educated me and given me solace and their efforts are to be applauded: AARP (AARP.org), Alzheimer's Association (ALZ.org), American Geriatrics Society's Health in Aging Foundation (HealthinAging.org), American Heart Association (heart.org), American Stroke Association (strokeassociation.org), BrightFocus Foundation (BrightFocus.org), Cleveland Clinic (My.ClevelandClinic.org), Harvard Nurses' Health Study (nurseshealthstudy.org), Health Reference Library (Healthline.com), Mayo Foundation for Medical Education and Research (MayoClinic.org), Medicare/Medicaid (Medicare.gov), Memorial Sloan-Kettering Cancer Center (mskcc.org), the National Insitutes of Health's Alzheimer's Disease Education and Referral (ADEAR) Center (adear@nia.nih.gov), National Institutes of Health's National Institute on Aging (nia.nih.gov), and the University of Illinois-Chicago, College of Medicine (medicine.uic.edu).

Second, these organizations should be praised for the eldercare and aging information that they provide on their websites: Eldercare.gov, Social Security Administration (ssa.gov), and the Virginia Division for the Aging (www.vda.virginia.gov).

Finally, I would like to recognize those friends, near and far, who were there for me at the hour of my need. Thank you.

Contents

Introduction

Your Story—Now

Today, or one day soon, you are going to have to start taking care of your parent and the Alzheimer's or other dementia that effects him or her. Maybe it starts with the after-work stopover you need to make to ensure that your mom's all right or to check that your dad's okay; the stop you make to ensure everything looks fine and the house is locked up for the night. Maybe you see the need growing from there. Maybe you're married with children and afraid it will challenge the time you have for those important family relationships. Maybe you're single and afraid it will interfere with your social life—after all, you decided you don't want to be single forever and finding the right person takes time. Maybe you're concerned that it will interfere with your job. Maybe you just can't move and give up your life at this moment to take care of your parent. Maybe you're too far away, in distance and in relationship, and you'll have to figure out how to surmount both your original problem with your parent and his current situation. Regardless of the circumstances, this book is for you.

My Story—How I Survived the Many Decisions, Twists, and Turns

My mother had multi-infarct (or vascular) dementia,[1] She was a registered nurse (RN), who graduated from nursing school when twelve-hour shifts assisting surgeons in operating theatres were not unheard of. Nursing, in all its facets, was her passion. She

---

[1] "What is Multi-Infarct Dementia," Healthline.com, accessed November 20, 2016, written by Lydia Krause, medically reviewed by University of Illinois-Chicago, College of Medicine on March 16, 2016, http://www.healthline.com/health/alzheimers-dementia/multi-infarct-dementia#Symptoms2 .

enjoyed the conversations with the patients; she enjoyed the challenges and intrica-cies of working alongside the doctors. As a registered nurse, she participated in the Harvard Nurses' Health Study[2]. The study followed over 100,000 registered nurses and was charged with assessing risk factors for cancer and cardiovascular disease. She felt it was important to help people understand illnesses, support those with medical con-ditions, push for more research and progress in areas where medical help may be lack-ing, and remove the concerns that cause people to hide their symptoms and issues. In line with that philosophy of contributing to health care, for over twenty-five years she shared her health and life experiences with the NHS and I shared her illness with them while completing the final study questionnaire that she would submit. Now, I am sharing some of what I learned from her illness with you.

Our family was lucky, because my mother, the nurse, told us what to do. She had decided early—when we children were actually just children—and told us often how she wanted any nursing or advanced care handled when she grew old and/or ill. She anticipated that at some point in her life she would need such care. Very thankfully, while she was well, she let us know that she wanted to be cared for at home, with nurs-ing care brought in, if necessary, and she (and my dad) made the financial arrange-ments that guaranteed that this setup would be possible. We kids and grandkids did as we were told. We didn't have the pressure to decide for her. She knew what she was saying and we were able to rely on her words.

Though I hope I have been discreet, I know that she would understand the inva-sions into her privacy that I have taken to explain or illustrate a point. I am equally assured that those close friends and relatives who survive her—those who knew what nursing and health care meant to her—will understand as well, and will gain from my candor on her behalf. Where I have trod too heavily, I hope she (as well as they) will excuse and forgive me, because this book is my contribution to her field.

I served as my mother's caretaker, assistant, companion, and friend for about sev-en years (and then spent about two additional years handling her estate). I somehow

2 "Harvard Nurses' Health Study History," The Harvard Nurses' Health Study (NHS), nurseshealthstudy.org/, accessed July 2017, http://nurseshealthstudy.org/about-nhs/history. The Harvard Nurses' Health Study began in 1976, charged with investigating risk factors for major chronic diseases in women. The study continues today, in its third generation, recruiting nurses and surfacing information to improve health for us all. Please access the NHS website for more information and tell a nurse about opportunities to join Nurses' Health Study 3 (NHS 3).

managed to do some of these tasks very well and to enjoy my parent's last years. Some things were hard for me, some things were easier, but nothing was easy. My first efforts were not that great, but I learned to do everything better. That is the key. The hard things I learned to keep trying until I could finally do them well. The easy things I learned to sustain, even when I was tired and didn't want to keep going. Stop thinking you're going to find the one solution, the one right way, and handle everything perfectly right from the start. That situation does not exist. You are going to bungle it at least a little, and hopefully with this book it will stay a little and not morph into too much. Still, there are some things I wish I had known before I set out. That's why I wrote this book for you.

This book is not an official this-is-how-you-do-it guide. It is a friend and companion on the often-uncharted road known as dementia. It will tell you some of the things you need to do and think about. It will also tell you that some of the things you're supposed to do—things you've been told will make your life better—are not going to go as planned, and you are going to have to dream up plan B, C, or even G. This book will help you know that's okay, you can still do a good job of caring for your parent (or other loved one), and more than that, you can do a good job of caring for yourself so that everyone goes through this stage and comes out the other end where he needs to be.

Your Story—Soon

If you are a person new to Alzheimer's and Other Dementia, you will learn about those illnesses, what separates them, and what can be done about them. If you're new to caretaking in general or to caretaking someone with Alzheimer's or Other Dementia in particular, you will learn some ways to do those things. If you're just beginning to tire from the load or are at your wits end, you will find out how to step back from that edge to a more pleasant and balanced life.

Learning from This Book and Listening to Yourself

When I was a kid, we used to play a game called "follow the leader," in which we would all hold hands, close our eyes, and follow whoever was in front of us. The leader at the very front of the line was usually some big kid who was good at talking people into doing stupid things. So, with our eyes squeezed shut, and with their eyes wide open, we would be dragged, serpentine-style, through the streets of the neighborhood. All of us kids would obediently comply, even though we were stumbling up and down steep yards, hitting our toes on curbs, bumping into telephone poles, and running into the odd fire hydrant. Eventually, our line would start to waver too much, and we would break our grips and fall on the grass—still laughing but relieved it was over. This was a great kids' game, but it is no way to go through life. *You are too old for "follow the leader." When it comes to your parent's care, follow your own good sense, your desire to protect your parent, and the real authorities in this field, who are out there. Do not just follow me!*

The questions, answers, statements, suppositions, and opinions in this book are neither all-inclusive nor written by a professional. Let my points and tips suggest questions of your own. Let them start you thinking of new and even better ways to adjust, cope, and triumph during what can be a trying time. I have simply put you on the path. It is up to you to decide in which direction you will walk. Take care of yourself, and after you make the trip successfully, let someone else know what you discovered so that their trip is even easier.

All my best.

How to Use This Book

How to Approach Reading This Book

Tip /tip/ noun
    A small piece of practical advice.[3]

chose "Tips" because you need something short, to the point, and immediately useful. That's what these thirty tips are. I am going to talk about how care starts and
how it ends, when to get help, where you might find that help, and when to run, not
walk, to the nearest exit and let professionals take over. Start where you need to start.
I have included both a table of contents and a "What Help Do You Need?" chart (see
below). They will guide you to the correct section to fulfill your specific caretaking
needs. For example, if you need to get your parent to stop driving, then start with Tip
15. If you need to decide where your parent will live, then start with Tip 16, then read
Tip 17 and Tip 18. If you need to decide whether you can do this at all because you feel
overwhelmed, read Tip 4, and then read Tip 26 and Tip 28. And most importantly, if
you need to get your siblings, husband, wife, significant or insignificant other, and old-
enough children on board, read Tip 27, then let them read a copy of this book. That
way, all of you know the ride you're going to be taking, whether you want to make the
trip at all, and if so, what you need to take with you to make it the best trip it can be.

---

3 Definition of the word "Tip," OxfordDictionaries.com, Oxford (English) Living Dictionary, Oxford
University Press, accessed August 29, 2017, https://en.oxforddictionaries.com .

Three Important Suggestions Before You Get Started

First, whether it seems out of your reach economically or in other ways, do not shy away from big-name hospitals, research centers, or other facilities. These organizations are the very ones that have the endowments and contributions needed to support important research, and often they can help you in accessing the best and most useful treatments. Ask for their assistance. That's why they exist, *for you*, not just for someone else.

Second, when it comes to accessing and using any of the Alzheimer's, dementia, or other websites indicated in this book, always be discreet with your personal information. Whenever you access a website be very aware that if you enter any personal information online it is out there and may be out there for quite a long time. Others, both official (and possibly unofficial) *will* access it. Therefore, always be thoughtful, cautious, and prudent about what information (medical, personal, occupational, etc.) you choose to share and include, and always err on the side of providing *less* information, not more. If an organization's website cannot help you without your providing tons of personal information online, then do one of three things: 1.) call them and give them the information by telephone, 2.) ask whether you can print out the online forms, fill them out offline, and mail them in (very old fashioned, but still affordable and reliable), and 3.) go to another website and see whether or not you can get the help you want there (and don't be too discouraged, professionals that will help you the way *you need* to be helped are out there).

Third, do not defer to my opinion when it comes to suggestions regarding your parent, rather, always look at any suggestions in light of how confident and comfortable you yourself feel about it. Judge all suggestions by how well they will work for your parent, not somebody else's. Some of the sources of further information (websites, etc.), companies referenced, or products listed may work for you and be a good choice; some may not. By listing them here, I am suggesting a place for you to *begin*, not end. Only access, consider, and/or try those things you yourself have checked out and found worthy of your time, money, faith, and participation. Use your own guidelines for what is appropriate for your parent at all times.

What Help Do You Need?

The table that follows lists each tip and what it has to offer you. It will help you find where you need to look in this book.

Tip	Where Should You Look If . . .
Introduction	If you want to know why I wrote this book and what I hope it will do for you
Tip 1	If you need to learn what the start of Alzheimer's or other dementia can look like and begin learning about the signs and symptoms
Tip 2	If you want to learn more about Alzheimer's and other types of dementia
Tip 3	If you need to find a doctor for your parent or want to know how to find out about new medications or treatments
Tip 4	If you want to think about whether you can (or should) take this on, or you need to decide whether you (or someone else) should take care of your parent
Tip 5	If you want to make sure your parent has the technology (and skills) he needs to help himself in his everyday life (e.g., home security system monitoring, vehicle monitoring, easy to use cell phone, useful emergency contact information with him at all times)
Tip 6	If you want to make sure that you have the technology to monitor your parent's well-being (e.g., monitoring location, cell phone activity, online activity, and home security)
Tip 7	If you want to make sure your parent's home is well setup to make his life easier now and/or you need to arrange to handle your parent's home improvements, parent's home maintenance, or home services
Tip 8	If you want to make sure your parent maintains social contacts
Tip 9	If religion or faith is important to your parent
Tip 10	If your parent has or needs a bank account
Tip 11	If your parent has or needs a safe deposit box
Tip 12	If you're concerned that your parent needs to be protected from fraudulent individuals

Tip	Where Should You Look If . . .
Tip 13	If your parent needs life insurance to protect his family, or to payoff outstanding debt or final expenses
Tip 14	If your parent needs to set up a power of attorney for medical (health care) and/or financial decisions while he is living, should he become incapacitated
Tip 15	If your parent still drives, whether it is a concern now or not
Tip 16	If you need to start thinking about more advanced care for your parent
Tip 17	If you and your parent need to consider ways to pay for your parent's care
Tip 18	If you need to select a care option and/or a housing/living option for your parent
Tip 19	If you need to learn about twenty-four-hours a day, seven-days a week (24/7) care
Tip 20	If you need to learn about hospice care
Tip 21	If your parent needs to stay in the hospital
Tip 22	If you need to know what to do if your parent goes missing, or you wonder about Silver Alerts
Tip 23	If your parent will need to divide his belongings among you and his other children and you'd like to see family valuables and family relationships maintained
Tip 24	If your parent needs a will (last will and testament)
Tip 25	If your parent needs to make final (funeral or memorial service) arrangements
Tip 26	If you find that you just cannot be there with your parent

Tip	Where Should You Look If . . .
Tip 27	If you need to come to a caretaking agreement with your siblings or other relatives
Tip 28	If you need to take better care of yourself
Tip 29	If you need to prepare for when your parent passes away
Tip 30	If you need help knowing what to do after the funeral or memorial service
Epilogue	If you need to find a way to think about all you have been through after your parent is gone

I'm not an expert, except by personal experience, and my personal experience has given me lessons in what to do and what not to do that I could not earn, get, find, or discover anywhere else. But still, this is just one person's experience—and a somewhat weary person at that.

By reading this book, you will know that what you are going through is normal, and for reasons none of us may know, necessary. No one who has not experienced a parent with dementia can begin to know what you are talking about and how it is effecting you. So, lean on the people who know and teach the people who don't, because they may find themselves in your shoes in ten or twenty years. It is best that they know what the destination is like before they get there. Take care of yourself, and let me know how it goes for you.

My journey was scary, maddening, funny, touching, deep, and trite. I both wish I had never done any of it—and I would not have missed it and being with my mother for anything in the world. I hope this book will make your journey easier and simpler. Just remember: caretaking will never truly be easy, and as with most things in life, it is never simple.

Good luck to you.

PART 1

The Alzheimer's or Other Dementia

How to Start

- Pay Attention to the Signs of Alzheimer's and Other Dementia

- Learn More about Alzheimer's and Other Dementia

- Find Out about New Medications and Treatments

- Decide whether You Can or Should Really Do This Caretaking

TIP 1

Pay Attention to the Signs of Alzheimer's and Other Dementia

How It Begins—Signs

t starts different ways. You're having a conversation with your parent and suddenly he utters something odd, or she does the strangest thing. You pause. You notice it, but you tell yourself he must have misunderstood what you just said, or she is just in an odd mood today. When this happens, if it happens to you, start being alert and notice what happens from this point on. You may be witnessing the signs and symptoms of Alzheimer's or other dementia. You may also be witnessing the beginning of your caretaking journey.

Know Typical Signs and the Alzheimer's or Other Dementia Symptoms They Indicate

- If your parent wakes up in the middle of Saturday night and starts to cook the breakfast that she would normally cook on a weekday at six in the morning, this might be a sign that she is **disoriented** when it comes to the date and day of the week, i.e., **to time**.

- If your parent drives to the same drycleaners he's driven to most of his life, but this time the road seems strangely unfamiliar and he feels lost, this might be a sign that he is **disoriented** when it comes **to place**.

- If your parent has not had an accident or other intervening event that has effected his motor skills and the use of his fingers, hands, or arms, and yet he can no longer sign his name to his checks, or if your parent is window shopping with you in the mall then suddenly seems agitated, confused, or uncomfortable about her surroundings, these examples might be signs indicating a **problem with thinking**.

- If your parent operated a microwave without even thinking about it, but now that same microwave is too much for him to figure out and the familiar task of reheating a meal is too difficult, or if your parent *frequently* forgets appointments, faces, names and the like, these examples might be signs indicating **memory loss**.

My Sign

My journey began with my mother's first major health incident. It's the event that I recall most often; it's the one that reminds me how easily changeable life is. Here's how it happened for me.

On a June or July afternoon, I came home to a peaceful house. I laid my McDonald's® meal in front of me. I expected that my mother—with whom I had moved back in after returning from living out of state for a few years—was simply off doing something and would be home in a little while. In the meantime, I would have a moment of peace and my favorite TV show. After I had finished my meal and had my fill of silence, I began to wonder where my mom was. I figured she had stopped by the grocery store or was out having lunch with someone. This was at one in the afternoon. By four, I began to worry. Normally, she would have returned home by two or two thirty. By five thirty, I was getting concerned. At about seven thirty, I started calling people. By eight, my list of calls included the local and state police. By eight thirty, I had called a relative and was in her car driving around, canvasing the area where we lived. We drove to all of the places my mother might be. Then I started thinking. Maybe she had a flat tire. Maybe she was ill. Maybe she could not get to a phone and was hoping someone would happen by and help her. At about nine or nine thirty, while still riding around, a policeman called my cell phone and let me know that my mother was all right, but that I would need to come and pick her up.

Her car had run out of gas earlier that day—when she had tried to make a trip into the city, to a location that I had asked, actually begged, her not to go to on her own. She had been driving around all those hours trying to find her way back home. She was not in an area where she drove every day, but she *was* in an area where she had been driving throughout her life. After many hours, she had been sitting in that car hoping someone would come by to help her. And finally, someone did: a police squad car that just happened to be patrolling the area. If it hadn't happened by, I'm not sure what would have happened to my mom. Given where she was—deep in a very large park, the size of some small towns—no one else probably would have happened by. No one good, that is.

When I walked into the station, I looked over at my mother, and for the first time in my life, she seemed smaller than me. When I walked over to her and hugged her, I knew it was time for me to start looking out for her.

The following day, I took off work, bought a gas can, filled it with five gallons of unleaded, and my mom and I headed back to the spot where she had left her car. The plan was to put a little gas in it, follow her to the nearest gas station, fill up her gas tank, and then the two of us would drive our two cars back home. At the time, I was still thinking that it was just the fact that some time had passed since she had driven in that area, and new buildings had changed the landscape. But when she had trouble following me on the usual route, and we began to hold up traffic with our twenty-mile-per-hour speed, I knew it was something more.

With the slow speed, cars began passing her and getting between the two of us to the point that I lost eye contact with her in my rearview mirror. I had made sure that her cell phone was turned on, that she had the earphone snug and secure in her ear, and that she would expect a call if we got separated. We had talked about it. So, I tried calling her on her cell phone. She didn't pick up. Then she picked up and set the phone down, but she never disconnected the call. I started yelling into my phone, hoping she would hear me, even if the phone was resting in her lap. She didn't. I reassured myself that she would know to pull into the slow lane and just take her time the rest of the way home. She didn't. I got home and hoped she would get there too. But, she didn't. She was lost again, and I started calling the police again. This time, I knew who to call. I called the station where she had been the night before. She wasn't there, but the police would keep an eye out for her and send a car to look around; I contacted a neighboring state's police department, since she could have crossed a state line by then. Within a half hour, I had two state police and two county police stations looking for her. Eventually, thank God, one of them called.

It was a different police station from the one the night before. This time when I walked in, the officer commented that she seemed confused. My mom and I walked out together, and I got us home safely. I accidentally on purpose "lost" her keys in a filing cabinet that night. I apologized to her the next day for being so clumsy with her keys and offered to drive her anywhere she wanted to go. (In hindsight, I don't really think she believed me when I told her that I lost her keys, but she went along with it anyway and for that I was grateful. I think she did so because what happened with her driving scared her too.) That was the day I became my mom's caretaker. There had been no warning signs of illness. I was as surprised by events as she was, but there we were nonetheless. That was where my journey began, and it continued in one form or another until my mom passed away and her estate was settled some nine years later.

Understand What These Signs Should Mean to You

I wondered whether or not to share this part of her journey with you. I decided to do so, because we all tend to brush the dementia's warning signs away. When things like this happen, we tend to say "Mom's just getting a bit older; there's nothing really wrong," or "Dad just didn't recognize our new house; he's only been here half a dozen times," but we need to learn to say, "There may be a serious health problem here; I'm calling the doctor."

Though what I've described seems easy enough to recognize now, things are not always what they seem. At the time, I didn't see what was really happened at all. I rationalized the first event. I had never been inside a police station before. When I walked in, my mom did not appear disoriented or confused. She knew what happened; thus, there was no memory loss. So, at the time, I vowed to make sure my mom's gas tank was always filled and a cell phone was always with her. That was initially all that I thought was needed and I was shocked at the event that followed (her getting lost again).

Here's the problem: The day before this incident, as well as the day after it, my mom could still enjoy a regular conversation with me or with others, go shopping with me, cook, answer the phone, respond normally to peoples' questions, and perform all of her other activities just as she always had. Even at the end of her life, when her dementia was advanced, she could still remember, communicate, and recite information. She enjoyed a Tom Selleck Jessie Stone movie marathon with me and knew who the actor was. She would sing along with the big band music she and my dad had danced to when they were young and get the lyrics right. She even followed mass on the television and recited all of the words to the Lord's Prayer correctly. Alzheimer's and other dementia can be mysterious in that way. One moment your parent is there and functioning highly. The next moment, or maybe the next week, they're not doing as well, then they're back again. They are themselves again. This is why we sometimes miss or dismiss the signs of Alzheimer's or other dementia.

Understand What You Should Do When You See These Signs

- Always, if you see odd behavior like that described above, **take your parent immediately to an emergency room or immediately to your parent's regular doctor's office, if it is near.**

- Tell them that your parent is experiencing unusual memory loss, disorientation to time or place, problems thinking, and anything else you observe. **Ask them to exam your parent.**

- Tell the staff there that you are concerned that a minor stroke, or other event has occurred.

- Listen to whatever advice the emergency room doctor and nurses tell you at the hospital, but also call your parent's regular doctor while you are waiting, and in addition, follow up with that regular doctor, either right after the emergency room visit or as soon as possible afterward. When you reach the doctor's office, tell them that it's an emergency-need-to-get-in-to-see-the-doctor-right-away issue, not a next week kind of issue. Do not allow them to schedule you for a few days or weeks away.

- Be careful of doctors who tell you it's nothing, that it's something but nothing can be done about it, and/or that there's no reason to try to do something about it. Follow any immediate care order as necessary, then, as mentioned, go to your trusted and well-known doctor. He or she will steer you from there.

It happens this way and it happens other ways. You need to learn about this issue and many other things in order to be of the most help to your parent. (And when I say "parent," I not only mean your mom or dad, I mean your grandparent, your uncle, your aunt, your adult friend. So, look out for them too.) Start your journey here and learn about Alzheimer's and other dementia.

TIP 2

Learn More about Alzheimer's and Other Dementia

Before You Begin

Must you learn as much as you can about Alzheimer's and Other Dementia? Yes and no. Learn as much or as little as is comfortable for you. It's okay to let the doctor be the expert, and it's equally okay for you to become one yourself. Take care of yourself during this learning process.

How to Understand the Difference Between Alzheimer's, Other Dementia, and Something Else

Alzheimer's versus Dementia

First, you need to understand that Alzheimer's and Dementia *do not* mean the same thing. Next, you need to thoroughly understand what each term *does* mean.

What Is Dementia? A General Definition

Let's start with dementia. Dementia is both 1.) the symptoms themselves and 2.) a category of diseases and conditions that produce these symptoms. When we are talking about dementia symptoms, it might help to think of dementia as *how you describe* what you see, as opposed to the cause of what you see.

For example, you might say (describe) someone as having a loss of memory, disorientation, an inability to perform certain tasks, that description—that is, someone having any or all of those symptoms—is what we call dementia.

Examples of dementia symptoms are what is being described in the situations listed in the typical symptoms section in Tip 1. The causes of the dementia symptoms listed are not stated. Furthermore, the fact that these symptoms could possibly be showing the presence of some other health concern rather than dementia is also not stated.

What Is Alzheimer's? A General Definition

Alzheimer's is a disease. It occurs when "abnormal deposits of proteins form [things called] amyloid plaques and tau tangles throughout the brain, and once-healthy neurons stop functioning, lose connections with other neurons, and die."[4] As a disease, Alzheimer's is *a cause of* certain symptoms. When Alzheimer's disease occurs, we see the memory loss and other symptoms that are known as dementia. Though we usually only hear about Alzheimer's, Alzheimer's disease is *only one of several diseases or conditions that cause or lead to the symptoms of dementia.*

What is "Something Else"? A General Definition

Something Else indicates that there are types of memory loss, and the other symptoms listed above, that are neither Alzheimer's disease, nor even related to dementia. These non-Alzheimer's, non-dementia-related symptoms have several possible causes that are discussed later in this tip, in the section on dementia-like conditions that can be reversed. Therefore, *do not assume* that everything you see, every memory slip or glitch, is Alzheimer's or other dementia. Do not make the mistake of concluding that every time your parent loses his glasses, misplaces the remote, or gets lost on the road you are seeing Alzheimer's or another form of dementia. It may be nothing at all or it may be something else.

---

4 "Alzheimer's Disease Fact Sheet." NIA.NIH.gov, Alzheimer's Disease Fact Sheet, Alzheimer's Disease Education and Referral (ADEAR) Center, National Institute on Aging (NIA), The National Institutes of Health (NIH), accessed July 19, 2017, https://www.nia.nih.gov/alzheimers/publication/alzheimers-disease-fact-sheet.

What Is Alzheimer's? A More Detailed Definition

When it comes to modern health care, most of us have heard about plaque and how it hardens the arteries contributing to heart disease. Alzheimer's disease involves plaque and a hardening process as well. In fact, according to the **BrightFocus Foundation**, and as noted above, "one of the hallmarks of Alzheimer's disease is the accumulation of amyloid plaques between nerve cells (neurons) in the brain."[5] BrightFocus Foundation goes on to say that "in a healthy brain, these protein fragments are broken down and eliminated. In Alzheimer's disease, the fragments accumulate to form hard, insoluble plaques."[6]

The **Alzheimer's Association** (ALZ) says, "Alzheimer's disease accounts for 60 to 80 percent of dementia cases."[7] *Alzheimer's is not a normal part of aging*, although the greatest known risk factor is increasing age. Although the majority of people with Alzheimer's are sixty-five and older, up to 5 percent of people with the disease have early-onset Alzheimer's (also known as younger-onset), which often appears when people are in their forties or fifties.

What Is Dementia? A More Detailed Definition

I have included three definitions of dementia. Two of the definitions are from leading United States medical institutions: The Mayo Clinic in Rochester, Minnesota (MayoClinic.org, Mayo Clinic's award-winning website, offers consumer health information) and The Cleveland Clinic in Cleveland, Ohio (My.ClevelandClinic.org is one of the top sites for health-related articles). The third definition comes from the Health Reference Library and was published by one of the leading organizations supporting health and wellness for adults 50 years old and beyond, AARP.

The **Mayo Clinic** lists the following definition of dementia:
Dementia isn't a specific disease. Instead, dementia describes a group of symptoms affecting memory, thinking, and social abilities severely enough

---

5 "Amyloid Plaques and Neurofibrillary Tangles." BrightFocus.org, BrightFocus Foundation, Alzheimer's Disease Research Program accessed July 27, 2017, http://www.brightfocus.org/alzheimers/infographic/amyloid-plaques-and-neurofibrillary-tangles.

6 Ibid.

7 "What is Alzheimer's?" ALZ.org, Alzheimer's Association, accessed November 20, 2016, http://www.alz.org/alzheimers_disease_what_is_alzheimers.asp.

to interfere with daily functioning. Though dementia generally involves memory loss, memory loss has different causes. So memory loss alone does not mean you have dementia. Alzheimer's disease is the most common cause of a progressive dementia in older adults, but there are a number of causes of dementia. Depending on the cause, some dementia symptoms can be reversed.[8]

http://www.mayoclinic.org/diseases-conditions/dementia/home/ovc-20198502

The **Cleveland Clinic** defines dementia this way:

When loss of mental functions—such as thinking, memory, and reasoning—are severe enough to interfere with a person's independent daily functioning, they are said to be at the stage of dementia. Dementia is not a disease itself, but rather the total impact of symptoms that might accompany certain diseases or conditions on daily function. Symptoms also might include changes in personality, mood, and behavior.

Dementia develops when the parts of the brain that are involved with learning, memory, decision-making, and language are affected by any of various infections or diseases. The most common cause of dementia is Alzheimer's disease, but there are numerous other known causes. Most of these causes are very rare.[9]

https://my.clevelandclinic.org/health/articles/types-of-dementia

---

8   "Dementia Overview," MayoClinic.org, Mayo Foundation for Medical Education and Research, accessed November 20, 2016, http://www.mayoclinic.org/diseases-conditions/dementia/home/ovc-20198502.

9   "What Is Dementia," My.ClevelandClinic.org, Cleveland Clinic Foundation (CCF) Health Library, accessed November 20, 2016, https://my.clevelandclinic.org/health/articles/types-of-dementia.

AARP's Health Encyclopedia sites the Health Reference Library as saying the following:

Dementia is a decline in cognitive function. It may affect memory, thinking, language, judgment, and behavior.[10]

http://healthtools.aarp.org/health/dementia-test-and-diagnosis-testing

What Are the Types of Dementia?

When I say "types of dementia," I am referring to a variety of different diseases, illnesses, and conditions that can cause or lead to dementia symptoms. So, when I ask, "What type of dementia does your parent have?" I am asking, *why is dementia present*? Which disease, illness, or condition has caused or lead to his dementia? As discussed previously, dementia symptoms are the thinking, reasoning, and orientation changes that we observe. Thus, three people may exhibit dementia symptoms such as memory loss, but one person's symptoms might be caused by Alzheimer's disease, the second person's symptoms might be caused by vascular dementia (which you will read about below), and the third person's symptoms may be caused by something else entirely. Therefore, if someone says his parent has dementia, you may understand *what symptoms* his parent is showing, however, you still will not know *why*.

Here are some of the currently known types of dementia. Links to both the Alzheimer's Association and the Mayo Clinic[11] websites are included to give you a sampling of the information available. Please note, that both the Alz.org and MayoClinic.org websites are extremely useful and will educate and comfort you. Follow the links and read the definitions with the idea that there are treatments available:

- **Alzheimer's disease**
  As the most common type of dementia, Alzheimer's is the one illness whose name is most often used, even for those ailments that are actually other forms of dementia or non-dementia conditions. Read more at the links below: (http://www.mayoclinic.org/diseases-conditions/dementia/symptoms-causes/dxc-20198504) (http://www.alz.org/dementia/types-of-dementia.asp#alzheimers)

- **Vascular dementia**
  Vascular dementia is another common type of dementia. Both the American Heart Association (http://www.heart.org) and the American Stroke Association (http://www.strokeassociation.org) discuss dementia and connect it those illnesses. Please access the Heart Association and Stroke Association websites and search for "dementia diagnosis" for more information and clarification. Also, read more at the links below: (http://www.mayoclinic.org/diseases-conditions/dementia/symptoms-causes/dxc-20198504) (http://www.alz.org/dementia/types-of-dementia.asp#vascular)

  In addition, read about transient ischemic attacks and their connection to this cause of dementia at the following link: (http://www.strokeassociation.org/STROKEORG/AboutStroke/TypesofStroke/TIA/Transient-Ischemic-Attack-TIA_UCM_492003_SubHomePage.jsp)

- **Dementia with Lewy bodies (DLB)**
  This is one of the more common types of progressive dementia. Read more at the links below: (http://www.mayoclinic.org/diseases-conditions/dementia/symptoms-causes/dxc-20198504) (http://www.alz.org/dementia/types-of-dementia.asp#dlb)

- **Mixed dementia**
  Mixed dementia is dementia that includes signs not only of Alzheimer's disease, but also of vascular and Lewy body dementia. It is found more often in those 80 years and older. Read more at the links below: (http://www.mayoclinic.org/diseases-conditions/dementia/symptoms-causes/dxc-20198504) (http://www.alz.org/dementia/types-of-dementia.asp#mixed)

There are some conditions that may be linked to Alzheimer's or other dementia. Do not get yourself upset by the mention of these illnesses. Read the Alzheimer's Association website for a more involved and medical definition. Read the Mayo Clinic site for a basic and useful definition. Both of these websites, along with the other websites mentioned in this tip, put an enormous amount of information, suggestions for next steps, and resources in your hands. Go forward. See your doctor. Let the doctor get rid of your concerns or let him or her assist you in finding the medical help that you need. What you can do this week or this month might make all the difference.

- **Parkinson's disease**
  Many people with Parkinson's disease eventually develop dementia symptoms (Parkinson's disease dementia). Read more at the links below:
  (http://www.mayoclinic.org/diseases-conditions/dementia/symptoms-causes/dxc-20198504)
  (http://www.alz.org/dementia/types-of-dementia.asp#parkinsons)

- **Frontotemporal dementia**
  Frontotemporal dementia is a rare form of dementia. Read more at the links below:
  (http://www.mayoclinic.org/diseases-conditions/dementia/symptoms-causes/dxc-20198504)
  (http://www.alz.org/dementia/types-of-dementia.asp#frontotemporal)

- **Creutzfeldt-Jakob disease**
  This disease is related to the brain, spine, and nerves. Read more at the links below:
  (http://www.mayoclinic.org/diseases-conditions/dementia/symptoms-causes/dxc-20198504)
  (http://www.alz.org/dementia/types-of-dementia.asp#creutzfeldt-jakob)

- **Normal-pressure hydrocephalus**
  The Mayo Clinic lists this condition as one of the dementia or dementia-like diseases that can be reversed. Access the mayoclinic.org website to find more information or read more at the links below:
  (http://www.mayoclinic.org/diseases-conditions/dementia/symptoms-causes/dxc-20198504)
  (http://www.alz.org/dementia/types-of-dementia.asp#hydrocephalus)

- **Huntington's disease**
  Huntington' disease has hereditary factors. Read more at the links below:
  (http://www.mayoclinic.org/diseases-conditions/dementia/symptoms-causes/dxc-20198504)
  (http://www.alz.org/dementia/types-of-dementia.asp#huntingtons)

- **Wernicke-Korsakoff syndrome**
  The Wernicke-Korsakoff syndrome is related to a lack of vitamin B-1 and its effects. Read more at the links below:
  (http://newsnetwork.mayoclinic.org/discussion/prompt-diagnosis-and-treatment-may-eliminate-symptoms-of-brain-disorder/) and (http://www.mayoclinic.org/diseases-conditions/dementia/symptoms-causes/dxc-20198504) (http://www.alz.org/dementia/types-of-dementia.asp#wernicke-korsakoff)

What is "Something Else"? A More Detailed Definition

Other Physical Conditions
There are numerous physical conditions, from dehydration to more serious ailments that can or might affect the memory. I am not qualified to discuss any of them, but the authorities I have cited in this tip are. Please read on. Consult the Mayo Clinic website (http://www.mayoclinic.org/) for more information on what is presented in this section and remember to take advantage of the helpful resources you discover there. Also, consider seeking out additional information on this issue from the other healthcare authorities cited in this tip.

Dementia-like conditions that can be reversed
According to the Mayo Clinic[12], some causes of dementia or dementia-like symptoms can be reversed with treatment. They include:

- Infections and immune disorders

- Metabolic problems and endocrine abnormalities

---

12 "Dementia-like Conditions That Can Be Reversed, Dementia: Symptoms and Causes," Mayo Foundation for Medical Education and Research (MFMER), Mayo Clinic, accessed March 13, 2017, http://www.mayoclinic.org/diseases-conditions/dementia/symptoms-causes/dxc-20198504.

- Nutritional deficiencies (such as vitamin B deficiencies—B-1, B-6, and B-12)

- Reactions to medications

- Subdural hematomas

- Poisoning

- Brain tumors

- Anoxia or hypoxia (<u>not</u> anorexia, but rather "anoxia," which has to do with a lack of oxygen)

- Normal-pressure hydrocephalus (which is also listed previously in this tip as a type of dementia)

I'm also here to tell you not to pretend any symptoms your parent does have will simply go away. Therefore, do not assume that you know what the problem is, that it's definitely dementia, or even that's it's simply that mom or dad is getting old. See a doctor. Tell him or her that you have concerns about memory issues. Say the words *Alzheimer's* and *dementia* out loud so that there is no issue of the doctor not understanding what you're concerned is happening. Then let him or her do the job of finding out what is really going on.

This book is about helping you start considering how to help your parent get care and set up the lifestyle structures that will keep him safe and well, now and in the coming years. Get your parent to a doctor. You do not know whether it is Alzheimer's, another type of dementia, or something else entirely. You, your parent, and your parent's doctor need to find out.

TIP 3

Seek a Diagnosis, Find New Treatments, and Maintain General Health

How to Seek a Diagnosis, Find New Treatments, and Secure General Healthcare

How to Seek a Diagnosis—Finding a Doctor Who Knows about Alzheimer's or Other Dementia

cannot tell you who to go see, but I can give you some suggestions on how to approach the issue. For instance, you could do the following to locate a doctor who knows about Alzheimer's or other dementia:

1. **If you have a doctor, start by seeing him or her**.

    o   Ask whether he or she can diagnose you himself or herself, or if he or she will need to refer you to (send you to) a doctor that specializes in Alzheimer's or other dementia.

    o   This actually may be necessary if your parent belongs to an HMO or other managed health care organization that requires referrals from the primary care physician in order to see a doctor for specialized care.

    o   **If you're sent to a specific doctor, then great. Move on to the next section to continue reading this tip.**

2. **If you don't have a doctor already (so you don't have anyone who can diagnose you himself or herself or give you a referral) or you prefer to select your own specialist—and your health insurance plan allows you to do so—then start here. to start searching for a doctor** with specialized knowledge of Alzheimer's and other types of dementia:

   ○ **Check whether your parent has Medicare coverage. If your parent does have it, then go to the Medicare.gov website and search for "Find Physicians and Clinicians."** Enter your or your parent's zip code, and select "Geriatric Medicine," "Gerontology," or something else for the type of doctor you prefer. Please note that at the time of this writing there is no specialty for "Alzheimer's" or "Dementia" available to select from the list.

   ○ **Consult your parent's medical insurance organization's doctors list for recommendations and search for dementia, Alzheimer's, or gerontology or geriatric.** These lists are provided—usually by a mailing to your home—in booklet form when you first sign up for your health care coverage. They are also provided at the insurance company's website. Look at the back of your insurance card either to find the member services number to request a new booklet or to find the exact website address so that you can access the information online.

   and/or

   ○ **Consult one of the following websites that specializes in Alzheimer's or Other Dementia information for suggestions:**

      – **AARP (AARP.org)** AARP has two new features, AARP States and AARP Dementia Friends, which I have not tried, but that you may want to check out:

         ○ **AARP States**
            Provides various links to resources in your state, some having to do with health and caregiving, others are more general: http://www.aarp.org/states/?intcmp=FTR-LINKS-INFO-STATE-EWHERE

- **AARP Dementia Friends**
  https://search.aarp.org/gss/everywhere?q=dementia%20 friends&intcmp=DSO-SRCH-EWHERE

– **Alzheimer's Association (Alz.org)** The Alzheimer's Association, which has offices in downtown Chicago, Illinois, has been mentioned several times, but here is its contact information again:

- **Alzheimer's Association**
  www.alz.org
  24-hour helpline, Toll Free: 1-800-272-3900

– **Alzheimer's Disease Education and Referral Center at The National Institutes of Health's (NIH) National Institute on Aging (NIA) (nia.nih.gov/alzheimers)** in Bethesda, Maryland, has an information clearing house that may seem a bit intimidating at first, but that is very useful. Here is contact information for both its National Institute on Aging and its Alzheimer's Disease Education and Referral Center:

- **Alzheimer's Disease Education and Referral (ADEAR) Center**
  Website: https://www.nia.nih.gov/alzheimers
  Contact: adear@nia.nih.gov
  Toll Free: 1-800-438-4380

- **National Institute on Aging (NIA)**
  Building 31, Room 5C27
  31 Center Drive, MSC 2292
  Bethesda, MD 20892
  www.nia.nih.gov

– **American Geriatrics Society's Health in Aging Foundation (healthinAging.org)** One of the best things about the American Geriatrics Society foundation's website, healthinAging.org, is their Tip Sheets. These brief information sheets cover topics such as how to obtain quality nursing home care, senior-friendly emergency rooms, and avoiding caregiver burnout.

o   **Health in Aging Foundation**
40 Fulton Street, 18th Floor
New York, NY 10038
Website: www.healthinAging.org
Call Us: 212-308-1414
Toll Free: 800-563-4916

–   **BrightFocus Foundation (BrightFocus.org)** The BrightFocus Foundation concentrates on research and finding a cure for brain and eye diseases, including Alzheimer's disease, (as well as Macular degeneration disease, and Glaucoma). They have useful information on both clinical trials and on the clinical trial process itself.

o   BrightFocus Foundation
22512 Gateway Center Drive
Clarksburg, MD 20871
Toll Free: 1-800-437-2423
Fax: (301) 258-9454
E-mail: info@brightfocus.org

3.   **Research doctors. Make sure to develop your own system. Here's one way that I do it:** First, of course, you search for doctors involved with dementia, Alzheimer's, gerontology or geriatric medicine and see what comes up. Second, when you get a list of possible doctors, simply be curious and read it. If there are photos, maybe you just like the look of someone, and think you would be comfortable around him or her. Accordingly, read his or her bio. Maybe you like the medical school that a particular doctor went to and so his bio catches your eye. Maybe another doctor's bio states that she is particularly interested in patients of your parent's age, and so that sparks your interest. Do they work at medical centers or in medical departments that are doing any special work in the field of dementia? If you read their bios or search their names, have they written any articles on Alzheimer's or dementia for any of the well-regarded websites? To me, these things show a

deep interest in the field, a knowledge of ongoing research, and a personal connection to their work—and thus potentially a good level of professionalism and concern for their patients. If you like ratings, when you find one or two names, look on websites that rate doctors and see whether or not they have complaints, and if they do whether those complaints are the "bad mix of personalities" kind or the "not a good idea to even explore this doctor" kind.

In addition, you could consider looking up local hospitals, particularly those associated with major research universities or those that advertise Alzheimer's or dementia care. Lastly, you could ask friends for recommendations of doctors that have helped them.

Make a Doctor's Appointment

First, make sure that the doctor you select can take care of you at the office/hospital you prefer. Doctors usually are associated with several hospitals in an area, pick a doctor that is already associated with the hospital you want to go visit.

Second, call the doctor's office, ask his staff whether or not he is taking on new patients. If he is, make an appointment for your parent. Also, ask the office staff whether they have a website where you can download, print, and fill out the usual new patient paperwork. If not, ask whether they can mail the forms to you to fill out. That way, you can fill them out a little at a time, in the comfort of your home, and you and your parent can discuss them along the way.

Before the Doctor's Appointment

Use the Doctor's Visit Form to Record Your Concerns

Prepare for your appointment. Before you get to the doctor's office, jot down the things about your parent's health that have been concerning you. I have included a doctor's visit form at the end of this tip. This form can be filled out as part of your preparation for going to the doctor. Let it help you to think of everything that worries you about your parent's condition. You can use it to hold detailed notes about your parent. You can also take it with you to the doctor, so that you don't forget your most important concerns. Let this doctor's visit form help you to have a more positive and productive doctor's appointment. (If your parent is at a more advanced stage, then consider also taking along the Assess Your Parent's Condition Checklist—see Tip 16. It might further assist the doctor in gaining a full understanding of your parent's current condition.)

Understand What the Doctor Will Do to Diagnose Alzheimer's or Other Dementia
According to AARP, "in April 2011, the National Institute on Aging (NIA) of the National Institutes of Health (NIH) and the Alzheimer's Association published specific criteria for diagnosing dementia."[13] Here are the typical steps AARP says the doctor will take when he or she is evaluating your parent for Alzheimer's or other dementia:

1. Gather your parent's Medical History

2. Give your parent a Physical Exam

3. Perform Neuropsychological Testing, such as the Mini-Mental State Exam (MMSE), which includes such thing as the following questions:

   ○ What day is it?

   ○ What time does the clock say?

   ○ Do you know where you are?

4. Perform Brain Imaging, such as MRI (magnetic resonance imaging) and CT (computerized tomography) scans used to help rule out brain tumors and blood clots, and PET (positron emission tomography) scans used to help see activity in the brain.

---

13 "What Do You Want to Know About Dementia?" Healthline.com, Health Reference Library, written by Wendy Leonard, MPH, published September 15, 2014, medically reviewed by Timothy J. Legg, Ph.D., CRNP, quoted in "Dementia Diagnosis," Health Encyclopedia, AARP.org, accessed November 20, 2016, http://healthtools.aarp.org/health/dementia-test-and-diagnosis-testing.

5. After you get your results, if Alzheimer's or another form of dementia is indicated, go the BrightFocus.org website. From their home page, click the Disease ToolKit link at the top of the page and select Alzheimer's. It will take you to an area where you can select and access their Getting Started Guide for managing a new diagnosis. Also, use the information that follows in the next tip.

After the Doctor's Appointment

Assess the Situation
If you find that you do not like the doctor for any reason, go back to your research and find another doctor. You need to feel satisfied with your choice, and that choice needs to be someone you can talk to and someone with whom your parent is comfortable.

How to Find Available Treatments and New Medications for Alzheimer's or Other Dementia

Read about an Old Approach (My Approach) then Consider a New (and Better) Approach
My Approach
Perhaps your experience is or will be different, but I did not have a great experience with the medical profession and getting my mother the care we wanted for her when it came to newly available medications and treatments. Let me explain. Both of my parents worked in hospitals most of their lives. Our family friends were doctors, nurses, hospital accountants, orderlies, and so forth. I used to trot down hospital corridors and see the clowns with the sick children who were on the ward. I used to run—sometimes a little too fast—to my dad's office when my mom drove in to pick him up from work. When I broke something, their friends put on my casts. So, I am neither afraid of nor intimidated by doctors. I like and respect most of them. Why am I saying this? Two reasons. First, because I do not want you to be too awestruck by doctors, nurses, and hospitals. Give them respect, but do not put yourself in a position "one down" from them so that you are listening to everything they tell you even when you know in your gut that it's not right or at least not the right thing for your parent at this time. Second,

I'm telling you this because I am someone who should have been able to navigate the medical system fairly easily, and yet, I found it difficult.

At the time, I was attempting to find out about trying a particular new medication for my mom, it was one that was being touted as a possible treatment medication for not only Alzheimer's patients, but also non-Alzheimer's dementia patients. I had hoped that—even though, like most non-Alzheimer's dementia patients, my mother's dementia had a physical cause different from that of Alzheimer patients, this new medication might help her. I made the appointments. I saw the doctors, but getting in to see anyone who would do more than suggest that I arrange for her to have more social time (at a senior center, for example) or have someone sit with her (when I was at work or otherwise unavailable) was very difficult. By the time I got to someone who *might* have actually helped by putting her on one of the latest medications at the time if he determined it was appropriate, the doctor said it was too late to do any good because of the stage of her illness. I cried. The problem was actually larger than I was. I had been trying to find out about and get my mom access to medications that might have prolonged her memory and her quality of life, but I was not able to do so primarily because of the particular type of or cause of dementia my mom had and also because of where research for dementia-related diseases and conditions was at that time.

If you find yourself in this situation, you will feel like you have failed. Why didn't you take him to the doctor sooner, some people will ask? (And they may not ask so nicely.) You know the answer: you did. You took him as soon as you knew something was up, as soon as you knew he wasn't quite himself, as soon as you knew there was a problem. It just wasn't good enough for the illness he has and the medications available cannot help everyone. If you find yourself in this situation, do your best. There are many things besides new medications that can assist your parent and help him to live out the best life he can if you find yourself in this situation. It may be the way you help them to continue the activities they enjoy for as long as they can. It may be in the care you do get for them, or the medication (drug) trial they are able to join.

Though, I do not have any good—which to me means tried and true—advice for you here, the rest of this tip includes suggestions that I hope will help you find a better way to approach this issue of new medications and treatments and find the help that you need.

A Better Approach

How to Start

Here is my best advice: if at all possible—for instance if you have a formal diagnosis long before more advanced symptoms begin to show themselves—start early to seek out information on new medications and treatments. Do not wait for your parent's condition to deteriorate. Now is the best time to start. Talk with the doctor. See whether he or she is up on the current research and is willing to help you find out about new medication protocols (new medication treatments, procedures, or guidelines) or clinical trials (the studies that help physicians try new medications and monitor their effectiveness). New medication protocols, or the clinical trials that test them, could give your parent a respite from some symptoms or may even buy him some time. Getting your doctor to advocate for you is probably the best way to enter this part of the medical system. You will need his or her medical expertise. You will need him or her to block for you if the people with the power of yes and no start to say no, which they probably will at some point. Keep talking to the doctor. Be kind but persistent until you are satisfied with the answers you receive. If you find that you are not being listened to, find a doctor who is a better fit for you and your parent.

Where to Start

While the doctor is your best and probably most reliable resource, you need to do your own research too. The better informed you are, the better it is for you, your parent, and your doctor. Doctors have unbelievable demands on them. Help them help you by becoming an informed advocate for your parent. Contact some of the resources indicated in this book— the Alzheimer's Association, the Alzheimer's Disease Education and Referral (ADEAR) Center at the National Institutes of Health's National Institute on Aging (which acts as a clearing house and includes information on many hospitals and other helpful organizations), and others—and find out about your parent's condition and about the latest clinical trials. These trials may be in your area or not. Do not let distance stop you from at least inquiring. A short trip could mean a difference in the quality of life for your parent, and you don't know what resources might be available to help you make that trip. If you find something that sounds good, show it to your doctor. Maybe he or she has heard of it. Maybe not. But either way, you can find out whether it is a possibility for your parent's care. Find out about other options. Find out about the latest research. Keep seeking information until you understand your parent's condition and feel comfortable discussing it. Keep asking, asking, asking—until you get the answers or information you seek. Polite is nice; getting the answer you seek is better.

As always, remember the caveat I gave you in the How to Use This Bok section, for all Alzheimer's and Other Dementia websites, be very aware that if you put personal information online it is out there and may be out there for a long time. Others, both official (and possibly unofficial), will access it. Therefore, always be thoughtful and discreet about what information (medical, personal, occupational, etc.) you choose to share and include. Always err on the side of *less information, not more.*

The Alzheimer's Association (alz.org) has something called Alzheimer's Association TrialMatch®. This online application will generate a list of applicable studies that your parent might be able to join. They have a video and step-by-step instructions to help you. Go to the following link: http://www.alz.org/research/clinical_trials/find_clinical_trials_trialmatch.asp to access TrialMatch® or call 1-800-272-3900 and press 1 for clinical trials). Accessing and using TrialMatch®, as with many of the databases mentioned puts you under no obligation to participate in their studies.[14] The Alzheimer's Association International Conference (AAIC), where diagnosis and a lifestyle trial were discussed. . (Abstracts from AAIC 2017 should be available in an upcoming issue of *Alzheimer's & Dementia: The Journal of the Alzheimer's Association.* Check out the AAIC website: http://alz.org/aaic/2017_news_releases.asp .

The Alzheimer's Disease Fact Sheet, Alzheimer's Disease Education and Referral (ADEAR) Center at the National Institutes of Health's National Institute on Aging has one of the best lists of hospitals to contact, many of which are conducting clinical trials that might be of interest. Access their website at: https://www.nia.nih.gov/alzheimers/clinical-trials or call 1-800-438-4380 (toll-free), Mon-Fri, 8:30 am-5:00 pm Eastern Time or send an e-mail to: adear@nia.nih.gov . They have a treatment map at the following link: It lists hospitals (what they call "Alzheimer's Disease Centers [ADC]") across the United States. In addition to their regular facilities, ADEAR's website states that some

---

14 Clinical Trials, Alzheimer's Association TrialMatch®, Alzheimer's Association (alz.org), http://www.alz.org/research/clinical_trials/find_clinical_trials_trialmatch.asp, access July 21, 2017.

of these centers have satellite facilities that are especially set up to assist underserved communities, rural communities, and minority communities.[15]

Use the BrightFocus Foundation to not only search for clinical trials, but to understand the clinical trial process better. Download a copy of *Clinical Trials: Your Questions Answered*: http://www.brightfocus.org/alzheimers-macular-degeneration-glaucoma/news/clinical-trials-your-questions-answered , then review the clinical trial information on the Search for Clinical Trials page: http://www.brightfocus.org/clinical-trials/search-clinical-trials .. Read more at their website BrightFocus.org or contact them by e-mail info@brightfocus.org or at 1-800-437-2423 (phone) or (301) 258-9454 (fax).

Also, access your state or local government via their websites and see what's there. Try using the AARP States link, it may save you time: http://www.aarp.org/states/?intcmp=FTR-LINKS-INFO-STATE-EWHERE. An alternative is to try searching your hardcopy phone book's government white pages. Many government offices now have centers for aging. Though current thought is that dementia is not caused by aging and that it is not a normal part of aging, age is often listed as a risk factor for the condition. Call your state or local officials and see what research or other options are available in your community. Government officials only know to earmark resources to certain parts of the community when they learn about the needs of the community. Make sure they know what you need. You might be surprised how that will help you and others like you in the future. There are many resources available now that were not available ten years ago, because local, state, and federal government, as well as private organizations and companies, have heard from their communities and have responded. By letting your needs be known, you advocate for your mom and dad, and you help someone else's mom or dad too.

You may also want to try a new website called TrialHero®, (https://trialhero.com/). TrialHero® is in partnership with Healthline.com, which is a health and medical news oriented website owned by Healthline Media. TrialHero.com provides an online form where you can enter your zip code and other information to locate clinical trials in your local area. At the time this book is being completed, they are advertising clinical trials for Alzheimer's Disease.

---

15 "Alzheimer's Disease Research Centers [ADC]," Alzheimer's Disease Education and Referral (ADEAR) Center, National Institutes of Health's National Institute on Aging, https://www.nia.nih.gov/alzheimers/alzheimers-disease-research-centers#statelist (accessed July 21, 2017).

These, as I said, are the best ways I can think of to leap this hurdle. Awareness has increased a great deal in the last ten years, and that should make your road a bit easier. Plus, you are more capable than you think. Remember, you do not have to be tough enough to fight through a Black Friday sale to do these things. Just do not expect everything to go perfectly, and be prepared to try and try again, if necessary.

How To Maintain Health Beyond the Alzheimer's or Other Dementia Diagnosis—Other Health Care Considerations

Maintain General Health Care

One last word on your parent's health: make sure that the doctor your parent sees is monitoring him for all of the symptoms appropriate for your parent's diagnosed condition(s) or refers your parent to another doctor to do so. What do I mean? If your parent has a heart problem, for example, he will need a doctor that monitors his heart health, not just his dementia (whether the dementia is related to the heart health or not). My mom was on medication that required that her blood and other indicators be checked regularly. I did not know this. Since she was handling her own health care at the time, I didn't learn about the monitoring from her. I learned about the need for monitoring from watching a TV commercial (a while after she had passed away) for a new medication that is meant to be better than her old one, primarily because it does not require such monitoring. The commercial said that lack of monitoring could lead to stroke. Small strokes, or TIAs (transient ischemic attacks), were one of my mom's health issues, and they could have increased the likelihood of the onset of dementia. I'm not sure how well she was monitored, and I wish I had known of the requirement from the beginning, while she was well and still functioning on her own. (She was off of that medication by the time her dementia was being handled.) Of course, I cannot be certain whether better monitoring would have made a difference to her health or not—sometimes nurses and doctors do not always take the best care of themselves—but I wish I had known. I would have made it my duty to make certain she got checked regularly. At least when she did come under our care, we kids were able to make sure she took care of herself and visited the doctor when she needed to do so.

So be annoying when it counts and make sure your parent has proper monitoring of all his medical issues. Remember that we all forget to take the best care of ourselves, and we all need a little someone on our shoulder saying, "I know you know what you're doing, but let's check with the doctor anyway." Know what checkups and monitoring your parent needs. If your parent won't record it on his calendar, keep it on your own calendar, and make sure your parent gets to his appointments.

Take Small Changes Seriously

Two times my mother woke me up and served me breakfast in the middle of the night. At 2:30 a.m., I got a knock on my bedroom door and a cheery, "Breakfast is ready." The first time, I felt too tired to get up, so I reached over, looked at the clock, and shrieked that it was too early and to go back to bed. The second time, having felt bad about the way I acted the first time, I got up and ate. Then I went back and lay down. No, she wasn't using her alarm clock, and that was part of the problem. She was used to being up, dressed, and in her car no later than 6:00 a.m. for years, and she was a bit too well rested and still naturally waking up early in her retirement. Perhaps, though, there was another issue there—a clue that her sleep pattern was beginning to change, that her body was off balance—and I didn't pick up on it. I dismissed it. So, make it a point to notice these little things. Write them down. Do not let a doctor tell you it's nothing or it's normal, because sometimes doctors will do that. Do not be a worrywart, but sometimes it's wise to sweat the little things. They could be the beginning of much larger things.

Form

ALZHEIMER'S OR OTHER DEMENTIA DOCTOR'S VISIT PREPARATION FORM

Alzheimer's or Other Dementia - Behavior Concerns

-

-

Alzheimer's or Other Dementia - Medication Concerns

-

-

General Health Concerns

-

-

Additional Comments or Questions

-

-

TIP 4

Decide Whether or Not You Should Be the One to Take Care of Your Parent

How to Decide Whether You (or Someone Else) Should Take Care of Your Parent

If you are still reading, you might need an aspirin by now. Believe me, it's not you. This is a lot, and it can be a lot for several years. So be sure you can do this—any of it—before you really begin.

Consider This If You're Already Worn Out

If you do begin and a voice inside says to stop, listen to it. Do not be stubborn and noble. Listen to it. If and when the time comes that you cannot care for your parent anymore, make sure that you have located the correct place and people to assist you. Do not bankrupt yourself. Do not give yourself heart palpitations, insomnia, or acid reflux. Know when to scream uncle. Give up when you've had enough—not five years after you've had enough—and allow your parent to be cared for by people who can change shifts and come to him fresh each day—and people perhaps better equipped to assist in those final hours. You must somehow keep thinking of yourself as number one in your life, especially if your parent means everything in the world to you. Your parent needs you sane and solvent. Do not be a hero for your parent and a coward for yourself. Your life counts too. Treat yourself as though it does.

Consider This If You're Trying to Honor Your Father or Mother, But Your Parent Was Not What You Needed

We are supposed to honor our father and mother. The Ten Commandments require it. People talk about it. Yes, I agree. Honor them. But what does it really mean to honor them? Does it mean to endure the parental abuse that we suffered as children because they now need our help? Does it mean to give to them when we have nothing left in us to give? I say no. It does not mean those things. And when it does start to mean those things, then what happens is that the mom or dad who is now feeble becomes our victim. Do not use my words to give yourself an excuse to hurt your parent. And do not tell yourself that you're doing something good because you deign to be in his or her presence. Stay away. Let others care for your parent. Send cards. Call. Visit, if that's appropriate. Give money or the items your parent needs (e.g., food, medical supplies, clothing—a nice new robe or jogging suit for him or her to lounge around in), but do not be there. Leave that to others. You may have an obligation to your parent, but how you fulfill that obligation does not have to look a certain way. Find your own way to honor your father and mother, by making sure he or she is safe, heard, and well cared for.

To me, honoring our father and mother means accepting them as God made them—appreciating their essence, comprehending the great people they are in some parts of their lives, and recognizing where they may fall short in other parts of their lives. It is not pretending we have perfect parents. It is appreciating that who our parent is, in all its forms, is important for reasons we may never understand. Nevertheless, we are not required to endure them or to denigrate the person God made us in favor of them. I believe that God wants both people to thrive.

One Last Word

There are many things in life that we think we're not up to handling. We lose sleep worrying and anticipating these things. Sometimes, though, these can be the very moments that make us greater than we are, that teach us things that other moments in life cannot. Bear this in mind as well.

Check out, and consider contacting, the organizations below before you make your decision. Still, make sure you make the best decision for you.

AARP Caregiving Resource Center
http://www.aarp.org/home-family/caregiving/planning-and-resources/

and also

https://search.aarp.org/gss/everywhere?q=AARP%20Caregiving&
intcmp=DSO-SRCH-EWHERE)

National Family Caregivers Association
1-800-896-3650
http://www.caregiveraction.org

PART 2

Your Parent

How to Use Technology to Assist Your Parent

- Make Sure Your Parent Has the Technology (and Skills) to Help Himself

  - Home Monitoring

  - Vehicle Monitoring

  - Cell Phone Usage

- Make Sure You Have the Technology (and Skills) to Help Your Parent

  - Track Your Parent's Location—Access Cell Phone Technology

  - Track Your Parent's Location—Access Vehicle GPS Technology

  - Track Your Parent's Call History

  - Track Your Parent's Online Activity

  - Monitor His Home, Inside and Outside

  - Monitor His Contacts with Neighbors and the People with Whom He Does Business

TIP 5

Make Sure Your Parent Has the Technology (and Skills) to Help Himself

How to Start Using Technology to Help Your Parent Protect His Home and Lifestyle

Get Home Security Monitoring for Your Parent

You can monitor a lot of things these days. You can set up audio and video to monitor the outside of his home, so that you have a visual and audio record of anyone who enters his yard, comes to the front door, or stands by the garage. In addition, you can set up monitoring throughout your parent's house.

Security Inside and Outside Your Parent's Home

People notice a lack of movement. They notice that no one comes outside the home, and the same car is always parked in the driveway and never moves. They notice that they don't see much movement through the curtains or that the light is only ever on in one room at the side of the house.

You could consider having someone active live with your parent, moving your parent into your home, finding another appropriate living situation as I will discuss later in this book, or you can use technology to help your parent's home to look and feel more lived in and secure. Consider some of these suggestions:

- Install switches to automatically turn on outside porch lights. Also, consider lights that line the walkway or the stairway and automatically come on outside when dusk arrives.[16]

- Don't forget the inside lights. Consider automatic timers for them as well, especially if your parent has a tendency to forget these.

- Install an appropriate security system, one that allows *you* to view inside and outside the home. Some systems allow you to turn lights on and off, check up on your parent's caretaker, see how well your mom or dad is doing that day, or look in on the cat or dog.

Read articles about home security. You might want to start with HGTV.com; it currently has an article online titled, *Aging In Place Home Technologies*. The link follows. The article focuses on home comfort and safety for those wishing to age in their own homes. The article has content from experts in home technologies and has great links to other important aging-related sites. Please read it (http://www.hgtv.com/remodel/mechanical-systems/aging-in-place-home-technologies). Talk to a security professional before you make any decisions. (And check with the Better Business Bureau [bbb.org], about the security professional or security company you contact.)

Get Vehicle Monitoring for Your Parent (OnStar®, Hum®, Zubie®, Automatic Pro®)

Another suggestion that I have seen used but have not used myself is OnStar® and similar services. If your parent is still driving, consider getting **OnStar** service or another vehicle-monitoring service for his car or truck. At this writing, OnStar is available on Chevrolets, Buicks, GMCs, and Cadillacs, including about thirty vehicle models. These monitoring systems can provide a calming voice to your parent and send emergency help or roadside assistance to them with the push of a button on the vehicle's dashboard or ceiling panel. These systems can also provide a vehicle location to police or emergency personnel under certain circumstances. Consider looking into one of these services. Call 1-888-466-7827 or go online to: https://www.onstar.com.

---

16 "Aging In Place Home Technologies," HGTV.com, accessed March 22, 2017, http://www.hgtv.com/remodel/mechanical-systems/aging-in-place-home-technologies.

There are other devices out there as well. Verizon® has a device called **Hum** (http://www.verizon.com/about/news/verizon-announces-availability-hum-creating-smart-connected-driving-experience-more-150-million). Zubie® has a product by the same name, **Zubie** (http://zubie.com/). Automatic Labs® has a device and claims it has zero fees; the device is called **Automatic Pro** (https://www.automatic.com/).

Some of these devices might be of more use on your end than on your parent's (the driver's) end, if they require that your parent be able to answer a cell phone in his car in order to say that he needs emergency services, instead of the device automatically sending an emergency service or providing a push button response system. Also, be careful of services that focus more on providing vehicle status information than on ensuring vehicle location tracking of your parent or expediting services to your parent's location. Therefore, make sure that the most important features function in a way that your parent can easily use them. You need to read the literature about these devices and you need to go see a demonstration of them to make sure that the features they talk about are the features you will actually get and your parent will be able to use.

Why is having easy access to vehicle tracking important? Because, as I mentioned earlier, when I called the police and reported that I thought my mother was missing, I asked about tracking her location I was told that a court order from a judge would be required. With these technologies, however, you have access to a convenient way to locate your loved one, quickly.

Get an Easily Useable Cell Phone for Your Parent

You could have a heart attack while you are the only one with your parent. He needs to be able to call for help and not be panicked and isolated. He could be out walking or driving and need assistance. Once again, he needs to be able to call for help when you're not there. I cannot stress this enough. This may be the most important thing that I tell you: help get your parent in the habit of always carrying a phone and make sure that he uses his phone frequently to stay in practice so that its use is automatic. Check out the Consumer Reports (consumerreports.org) article entitled *Best Smartphones for Seniors* (http://www.consumerreports.org/cro/news/2015/08/best-smartphones-for-seniors/index.htm) to get some ideas. A phone is useless if you cannot use it, for any reason.

Cell Phones—Make Sure Your Parent Has Some Kind of Phone or Calling Device
Smart Phones
Teach your parent to use a cell phone as soon as you can, and definitely while he or she still has the ability to retain the information. This is a big one. If your parent gets lost, he can still reach you and safety if he has a phone and knows how to use it. Let your parent start by using a regular phone. That way even if he has to borrow a stranger's phone he will have the skills to use it. If you want to buy your parent the popular iPhone (made by Apple) or a Galaxy (made by Samsung), great. Lay down the cash and buy it. I get it. I love them too, and for now, it may be just fine. If your parent loves technology and new gadgets, you will be a hero. Just make sure that he knows how to use that phone and make sure he always carries it with him.

Whether he's gardening in the backyard, out with his friends, or with you, your parent should have a phone with him (held in some safe fashion, such as on a belt loop or in a pocket).

Basic and Standard Phones
Another option is to get your parent a simple cell phone to use. Often, they are less complicated than the average smartphone. They sometimes have bigger numbers, so they are much easier to read and to dial, which can be important for people with vision problems, arthritis pain, or motor skill issues. Try Consumer Cellular (https://www.consumercellular.com/Products/BuyingGuide) for ideas on simple phones and some models that might work.

Special Call Devices
Yet another option, is an alternative style "phone" that commercials advertise as an "emergency-call button" that users can wear around their necks or sometimes on their wrists. For example, remember Life Alert's (http://www.lifealert.com) "I've fallen and I can't get up"™ ads? Well, that is the kind of alternative "phone" that is being discussed here. There are several companies that advertise products similar to this one. One that stands out is GreatCall's Lively Mobile®, (https://www.walmart.com/ip/Lively-Mobile-Urgent-Response-One-Touch-Waterproof-Device-by-GreatCall/54706754#about-item) sold at Wal-Mart Pharmacy. Lively Mobile's® spokesperson, John Walsh, created and hosted TV's *America's Most Wanted* and

spearheaded legislation on missing children. (The "Code Adam" that has been used in some Wal-Mart stores for children who go missing inside the stores while out shopping with their families is related to these efforts.) Though I have never tried either of these products, these two seem like a very good place to start in considering a different style phone for your parent. Though these products advertise their usefulness in various locations, take it upon yourself to find out for yourself whether the range is appropriate and its usefulness will fit your and your parent's individual needs. For example, will it work at your mall, your grocery store, your golf course? If it's just in the backyard, then your parent still needs a cell phone of some kind, and you still need to make it the easiest one for your parent to use. Also, test it in the places you might assume it will work, like your bathroom and basement or cellar, if you have one.

Though I have never tried either of these products myself, these are two that I would consider for my own use, after I performed the exact kind of further investigation that I am suggesting to you.

Remember, your parent *may not* remember how to use that smartphone and all of its buttons, but he *may* remember how to push that one button on one of the simple or the alternative phones, no matter what kind of day he is having. The chance of that is worth the price and the time it takes to find one of these alternatives and teach your parent to use it.

Prepare Your Parent's Cell Phone for an Emergency

Be Careful Using Passwords on Phones

Be careful about passwords on phones. A password may prevent your parent from using either their own phone or your phone in an emergency.

If there is a password on your parent's phone and he forgets it, his phone is all but useless. And it may not need to be a complicated password for him to forget it. We all forget things when we are rushed or upset. We also sometimes forget things due to our illnesses. In addition, they need to be able to access the call dialing keypad without going through a complicated menu. So, make sure that no password is ever put on the phone and the call dialing keypad comes up the minute you pick up the phone, or some similar safety feature is put in place. For help with this, see your phone retailer—and make them give you a demonstration before you take the phone home or go to the phone manufacturer's website for assistance.

One last thing, remember—as I have mentioned earlier—if you are alone with your parent and have a health emergency, it is your parent who might have to contact emergency help by dialing 9-1-1 (which they may remember because they have probably heard about it most of their lives). If that situation occurs and you have a password on your phone, your parent will be unable to use your phone unless you have a one button push way to by-pass the short or long password and access your keypad.

Setup Emergency Dialing on Cell Phones

Most phones can be setup to only require that the user push one button in order to speed-dial 911, to summon help to his location, or similarly to speed-dial your phone number. A one-button push is information that your parent may be able to retain and use in an emergency. Remember to set this up if it is not already setup.

Put Emergency Contacts and Information on Cell Phones (and on His Person)

You can also make sure your parent's phone contains a picture of you, as well as your phone and address contact information. If people cannot communicate well verbally, hospitals and police as well as fire and emergency medical services (EMS) rescue teams have been trained to review wallet and phone information to identify individuals. Make your parent's phone as good a communicator in the information it carries as it is when it can be used for calls. The American Automobile Association (AAA) has some great suggestions on what information is most useful to include. Check out the "cell phone ICE" (for AAA, ICE stands for "In Case of Emergency") information at their website, AAA.org (https://midatlantic.aaa.com/traffic-safety/cell-phone-ice). (By the way, as mentioned above, do not forget your parent's wallet. Make sure this information is there too. I made sure that my mom had identification on her in several places whenever she was with anyone else or even out with me.)

Maintain Continuous Cell Phone Service
Cell Phone Bills

Whether your parent uses a regular cell phone or one of the special types of phone, the phone bill must be paid and paid on time to maintain the service and for the phone to be of any use. Your parent may be on a fixed income. He may be too proud to ask you to help pay his cell phone bill. Be mindful of these possibilities. Pay the bill yourself, if possible, or make sure your parent has a low-cost, easy-to-maintain plan that will give him the phone service and protection he needs.

TIP 6

Make Sure You Have the Technology (and Skills) to Help Your Parent

How to Track Your Parent's Life

Track Your Parent's Location—in General

Why you're having easy access to location tracking is important for your parent and for you

At the beginning of this book I related a story about my mother's getting lost in her car. That day, when I called the police and reported that I thought my mother was missing, I asked about tracking the location of her cell phone, which she might have had with her. I was told that a court order from a judge was the only way that I would be able to do that. With the technology discussed below, however, that allows you to access cell phone location as well as vehicle location, you have access to reliable technology that allows *you* to locate your loved one, quickly.

Why you should be glad that officials are not supposed to just give out anyone's location

Now, before any of you get upset over the unwillingness of the police to use their resources to track my mother's cell phone location without a court order, please keep in mind that the police must protect not only your parent who may need to be found, but also those adults whose safety could be jeopardized if just anyone, at any time had easy access to their location simply by calling the police and asking for it. (Here, I'm referring to individuals who may be leaving an abuse situation and who rely on discretion, privacy, and even secrecy for their own safety and that of their loved ones.) So, keep this in mind, and get the technology needed to protect your parent and get it set up correctly by a professional.

Use Cell Phone Technology to Track Your Parent's Location

Though I suggest an easy-to-use phone for your parents, smartphones have good elder-care uses too. For example, if your parent uses an iPhone, with his permission, you can set up his phone to track his phone's—and thus his—location, if he has the phone with him and an appropriate Wi-Fi connection has been established. (It may be possible to monitor individuals using the basic- or standard-style phone described in the last tip, but you will need to check into that on your own.) While you're in the Apple Store, Best Buy, Walmart, Target, or any other major phone retailer, ask the knowledgeable salespeople there about the Find My iPhone or Find My Device app, then ask them to show you how that feature works—not just to tell you about it, but to *show* you how to set it up on the phone and use it, because things always *sound* easier than they actually are when you don't really know what you're doing. If the salesperson doesn't know how, ask him to find someone who does, or ask if the store has a class or workshop where these features are explained and demonstrated. I learned a lot at the Apple seminar I attended on the use of my computer. I'm sure that they, and other phone manufacturers and retailers, have classes, online instructions and tutorials, and other ways to teach you to use their products well. This could be very useful in preventing worry and making sure you know where your parent is and that he is safe. When my mother got lost in her car, this would have set my mind at ease and allowed me to reach her even if the police had not happened by.

Use Automobile GPS Technology Track Your Parent's Location

If your parent's car or truck has vehicle GPS technology (OnStar®, Hum®, Zubie®, Automatic Pro®), then you can be officially added to the list of people who can access this technology and gain location information for your parent. See the Get Car Monitoring for Your Parent section in the previous tip.

Track Your Parent's Call History

You can set up alerts on your parent's phone to notify you if and when calls are received from certain numbers. Review the instructions that accompanied his cell phone purchase or access this information online at the phone manufacturer's website. If the cell phone bill comes to you, you can also review the detailed bill for this information or go online to review the details. In addition, many cell phone providers allow you to go online to your account (in this case your parent's account) and block any unwanted phone numbers.

Track Your Parent's Online Activity

General Online Activity
You can monitor your parent's general online activity with the many parental-control applications and tools that are available on the market.

First, use the tools provided in the software already on your parent's computer. Both Microsoft (Windows) and Apple (Macs) computers have applications that allow you to set controls for individual user accounts that enable you to block access and limit computer usage.

Second, use the online monitoring software applications available on the market. Some were originally designed for monitoring the online activities of children and teenagers. To get the product that will work best for your parent's situation, after familiarizing yourself with the products out there, talk to your retail store expert about what you need. For starters, try going to CNET.com and searching for "online monitoring software." There you can add "Windows" or "Mac" to your search to find software for your specific computer. Lots of product suggestions displayed when I performed this search. To narrow your choices—and get a list of the best quality products—make sure that you also select Editor rating three-stars & up or four-stars & up, which will give you a list of the products that the CNET Editors consider best. Also, consider selecting the User rating three-stars & up or four-stars & up to help ensure that the products perform for the average user (you) as well as they perform for a computer industry expert (the CNET Editors).

Banking Online Activity
In addition, you can monitor your parent's banking if you are a signatory on his account, and therefore you can sign in to the account just as he would.

E-mail and Social Media Online Activity

Sometimes it's a good idea to monitor his online correspondence (whether in e-mail or on social media) so that you will know *before* he writes a check for $2,000 to that nice young woman he met online who wants to fund her own startup business, or before she says "yes, come on over" to that nice middle-aged man she met online, who offered to stop by and take some of your dad's old junk—that suitcase full of memorabilia that he hung on to most of his life and which he had planned to take to an antiques dealer for an appraisal—off her hands.

Monitor Your Parent's Home via His Home Security Monitoring System

You can use the monitoring devices set up in your parent's home, and discussed in Tip 5, to check up on your parent's home, and by extension on your parent. A door left fully open or even ajar, a dog not feed properly, a stove left on for hours, all of these are signs that perhaps more help, a homecare worker, or a change of housing/living may be needed. A delivered package that you see being picked up by someone else, a fence that keeps being climbed by neighborhood kids, might be an indicator that your parent's neighborhood is changing and that maybe it's time for him to leave and try something new. So, don't miss them. Don't just setup a security system, make sure use it fully:

- Check on whether that package your dad was expecting was delivered, handled properly, and left alone.

- Check on whether that package your dad was expecting was delivered, handled properly, and left alone.

- Check on whether your mom remembered to close the back door, or whether she stumbled taking the garbage out, but didn't tell you about it because she didn't want to worry you.

- Check on whether the cat got out when the lawn crew came in, or whether the house sitter left the dog outside in his kennel too long.

- Check on whether your dad's car really is being bothered by neighborhood kids or someone else really is trampling through your mom's flowers.

Also, once again, for more information read articles about home security. Start with HGTV.com's article, *Aging In Place Home Technologies*. (http://www.hgtv.com/remodel/mechanical-systems/aging-in-place-home-technologies).

Also, Remember to Monitor the Technology that Monitors Your Parent's Home
One last thing, remember that security companies are nothing more or less than people talented in technology and in how to use it to secure your parent's home. Do not just give them carte blanche to your home. Know who and what they are. Learn about any technology they install and understand what happens with that technology when you no longer want the service and need to restore your parent's home's privacy, either because someone else in the family will be living there or because you are selling home, for example (talk to a security professional about it). Make sure it continues to have the features you require and that the system is online and operating appropriately at all times.

Monitor Your Parent's Contacts with Neighbors and the People with Whom He Does Business
If your parent does not live with you, and you didn't grow up with the neighbors now living next door to and across from your parent, make a point to meet your parent's neighbors. Also, while your parent is still well, meet not only his or her new next-door neighbor but also the banker, insurance agent, lawyer, doctor, dry cleaner, massage therapist, newspaper carrier, mailman, hairdresser/barber, and any other professional with whom he does business. Do it as soon as possible, like now. Put down this book and start scheduling appointments. You have to know people. Period. There is no substitute for that. You need them to keep an eye on your parent. You want them to call you if bills aren't paid or your parent doesn't look good that day. If at all possible, they need to know what you look like, not just how you sound on the phone. And please believe me when I tell you that it is the only way you're going to get some things done. These individuals need to know and trust you. Plan extra time for a visit when you travel home for the next holiday. If you are too far away or don't have the money to travel, there's FaceTime, Skype, Go-to-Meeting, WebEx, and a host of other ways to make visual contact with the people in your parent's life. I have used all of these services at one time or another and have found them all to be reliable, helpful, and easy to use once you have a bit of orientation. Just remember to be security

conscious whenever discussing personal, professional, financial, or legal matters using these technologies. Also, note that fees, downloads, and other setup may be required.

For more information on the applications mentioned above, read the information below, then access the links provided:

- **FaceTime®**
  FaceTime is an Apple product (see Apple.com) that allows you to video chat (see and hear) with another person, regardless of their location. The application comes with the Apple iPhone. It can also be downloaded from the Internet. You can access https://www.apple.com to find out more about FaceTime or use this link for instructions with pictures on how to use it: http://www.wikihow.com/Use-FaceTime

- **Skype®**
  Skype also provides video chatting. At this writing, according to the Skype website, if you have Microsoft Office 365—which is when you access MS Office online through the Microsoft website rather than by purchasing the software at say BestBuy and using a CD to put the software on your computer—the service comes with 60 minutes of Skype time to use calling 60 country destinations. Access https: www. skype.com for more information

- **Go-to-Meeting®**
  With Go-to-Meeting you can even display documents, such as your dad's finances that you might need to discuss with his banker back home. https:// www.gotomeeting.com

- **WebEx®**
  WebEx also allows you to easily display and discuss information online. It's perfect for exchanging information with your mom's attorney. Just make sure to remember the need for caution and possibly additional security measures on your computer when having these discussions. https://www.webex.com

How To Improve Day-To-Day Life For Your Parent

- Maintain Your Parent's:

  - Home

  - Social Contacts

  - Religious Practice

TIP 7

Help Your Parent Maintain His Home

How to Handle Home Setup, Improvement, and Maintenance

This may be one of the most important things I say in this book, because it goes directly to the main issue here, ensuring that your parent can remain independent for as long as possible. Do repairs or renovations; get the home comfortable and up to code while your parent is well, then do not change the home.

Review Home Setup

Try to Keep Your Parent's Space as He Prefers, While You Make Sure It's Setup as It Needs to Be

Before you get started with improving and maintaining your parent's home, get clear about whose home it is and what the purpose of that space is: It is your parent's home (not yours) and it is where he expresses himself, where rests, and often the only place on earth where he can go and have peace on his own command.

Your parent knows his home—where the sofa is and which steps creak. He may not even realize how much he is relying on these cues rather than on his failing eyesight or his sometimes-unreliable memory. The minor act of moving the furniture around could cause issues for him. Be aware of this fact.

Also, your parent's home setup—the pictures of you kids on the table or wall, the old cabinet of your grandmother's that holds the holiday china, the beat-up

Barcalounger chair and the old TV trays in many ways that *is* him. (If you remember the TV show *Frasier*[17] and character Martin's old chair, pork rinds, and beer, then you know what I'm talking about here.) Please remember that. He may have spent more than half of his life in this space. Respect it and respect the way he keeps it. Do not just storm in with changes and improvements that may help, but in your parent's mind only make him feel sad, old, and out-of-control of his life.

Be Smart about Home Improvement

Before You Make Those Changes, Remember Small Changes Can Create Big Issues

If your parent has used the same microwave for three years, do not throw it out and get him that swanky new model. Why? Because he probably will not get much out of those great features you love so much. Maybe the writing on the dials is too small, or the operation instructions are too complicated. He may no longer be able to absorb the instructions on how to use a new appliance. By getting rid of the old microwave that he *does* know how to run, you may take away his ability to fix himself a hot meal or heat up a cup of tea. A sixty-dollar microwave gift for him just added the cost of a home caretaker to your tab, because someone is now going to have to cook all his meals and snacks for him. So, consider all of the consequences when you think about making household changes.

Arrange to Handle Home Maintenance

Get Your Parent the Home Help (Home Services) He or She Needs

Now that your parent's home is in order, get him the help needed to keep it that way. When I say home maintenance, I mean not only cutting the grass, dusting the house, and fixing what gets broken, I also mean buying groceries; preparing meals; purchasing personal care items; moving the cars around; and making sure lights and curtains are adjusted to suit the time of day and to communicate a lived-in home. Start by reviewing these questions:

---

17 "Frasier," 1993-2004 TV series, IMDb.com, accessed July 2017, http://www.imdb.com/title/tt0106004/releaseinfo?ref_=tt_ov_inf .

- What about inside the house? Is there someone who can dust and clean?

- If appropriate, can someone open and close the curtains daily. (Regarding curtains, please do not freeze your older relatives in the colder months by insisting that every curtain in the house be open to allow light in. Their old house probably has old windows that will leak as much heat as possible to the outside. Drawn curtains keep rooms warmer and they do it without costing a dime. Older people, especially those on fixed incomes, cannot afford to heat the outside, as your parent probably used to say.)

- Does your parent have a way to safely fix himself small meals when you or someone else cannot be there? If not, is it possible to get meals brought in, such as through a meal service like Meals-on-Wheels™ (LetsDoLunch.org) (or even through a service like Diets-to-Go, an online, national meal delivery service for those who might need to lose weight and cannot manage all of the special meal preparation or who might be on a doctor-approved Pre-Diabetes meal regimen). Remember that your parent's doctor must pre-approve any and all of these dietary changes, to make sure that something as simple as grapefruit added to a meal, for example, does not interfere with your parent's medication or treatment. Also, you could hire someone who can cook and serve meals daily, when necessary.

- What about pets? Is he able to feed and take care of a dog, cat, or other pet? Does he have enough money for pet food as well as occasional check-ups and grooming for the animal? Is there someone who is comfortable handling the pet who can come by daily and give the dog exercise or make sure the cat hasn't gotten into a space that it can't get out of on its own? Pets give us a lot. They help people—sometimes especially older people or those who live alone—live longer and happier lives. You need to make sure someone is there to take care of them.

- Does he or she require that groceries be ordered and delivered (so that driving and lugging heavy bags is avoided? In many cities and towns, you can now set up regular deliveries as well as shop online and have food delivered anytime you want. (Giant and Safeway grocery stores are among those store delivery services I have tried, and have been very happy using.) Also, many grocery stores now have personal shoppers, who will hand pick the groceries you order online and your parent can simply drive to the store, park in the designated spots, and have his groceries brought out to his car. Take advantage of these services. Their delivery fees are usually not expensive. Your parent can also do this from his own computer. Help him access it and set it up.

- If you buy groceries and/or personal care items for your parent have you considered what his or her current needs are and adjusted what you purchase or buy? Sometimes incontinence issues begin and worsen. Have you read the ads about such products that adults initially use—like those from companies such as Depends and others? Do you know that they have different product styles for men and women? Have you asked whether a company has progressively more protective products for use as your parent's condition progresses? Do you know which products must be ordered from a medical supply company and which ones can be bought in stores such as Costco or Wal-Mart, either in person or online? If you think your parent might be too embarrassed to ask you to purchase these products, then help your parent know how to order them him- or herself. He or she needs to know that they can be bought through online drug stores—such as CVS. com, Drugstore.com or Walgreens.com, through one of the large-box stores mentioned above, at the grocery stores that deliver like the ones listed or those in your area, or at special medical supply retailers online. Help your parent access these resources.

- What about the heavier jobs around the house? Is there someone who is *safe, reliable, and responsible* who can handle them? Is there someone who can shovel snow for your parent and make sure the basement does not flood during a bad storm, someone who shows up and does it and does not rely on your parent to track him down? Your parent will need someone to cut the grass and rake the leaves. Once again, it needs to be someone who shows up, does the work, and does not rely on your parent to find him.

- Can someone move the car around and take the trash cans in and out?

- Have you done a security check on anyone who will be around your parent in your absence? Cooks, caretakers, lawn services, etc., should all be thoroughly screened.

- Cable service, security system, and repair people should not be in the home unless you (or someone you trust) are there with your parent. Period. Otherwise, you may risk ending up with a security system or cable TV channel package that neither your parent nor you want or can afford, or a home repair bill that costs more than a new appliance might have. On top of the financial repercussions, you must always protect your parent's personal privacy and safety.

Do not forget that you will need to arrange a way to pay for the services that people render so that your parent does not need to negotiate with people or handle cash if he is uncomfortable with that.

Sometimes after you assess all those things, you may conclude, as children have done for years, that it would be cheaper, easier, and safer if your parent lived with you instead of on his own. If you do come to that conclusion, please read the tips on housing/living situations (Tip 16, Tip 17, and Tip 18) to help you start thinking about those issues.

TIP 8

Help Your Parent Maintain Social Contacts

How to Help Your Parent Maintain Friendships and Participate in Activities

While your parent is still well enough, help him maintain social contacts by re-establishing old friendships, meeting new acquaintances, and getting involved in new activities. Judge any activity by how well and how safely your parent can participate in it. Always ask yourself, whether your parent is well enough to be out on his own, whether others will be there to assist (and know to assist if your parent experiences any difficulties), and whether he is capable of getting himself to safety in any and all conditions that might arise in that situation.

Help Your Parent Participate in Established Activities with Old and Dear Friends

Help Your Parent Get Reacquainted

Start with your parent's current group of friends, if he has one. Often, we adults find it hard to maintain friendships while we work all day—inside and outside the home—and take care of our family lives, but if your parent has managed to maintain some friendships, encourage him to stay in contact with these friends. These are the people who will not only brighten his days, but also help him maintain his mental and physical functioning. We all need stimulation and friendships help us get it. For example, if your parent knows she'll be seeing her friends, she'll automatically make sure she can recount some stories to impress them, and keep up with the latest Hollywood or even neighborhood gossip so she can put her two cents in. Your father will make an extra effort to walk more, if his old competitor is striding two steps ahead of him when they meet.

If your parent is a homebody, find a way for him to have friends over and offer them refreshments, some sandwiches, salads, or a casserole for lunch. If fixing such a spread is too much for your parent, then consider another way. Order a platter of sandwiches from the deli counter at your local grocery store, make food and take it over yourself, or go over to his house the night before and help him make sandwiches or bake a casserole while the two of you chat. It's not a lot in the grand scheme of things, but it can mean happiness to your parent—and ultimately more peace of mind for you. Your parent needs time to chat with his friends about times that you're too young to remember. He needs time to gossip with relatives. He needs a life. People who aren't in the grave shouldn't act as though they are, no matter what their difficulties. It will make your parent feel better when he gets out of bed if he has something worthwhile to do.

If your parent had activities that he was involved in, but just hasn't been doing for a while, help him get back to them. Maybe he can still play chess or checkers down at the tables in the park. (If you don't feel comfortable with him being there entirely on his own, then maybe your parent can play while your kids run around with their friends and you read a book.) Maybe he can still jog with his running group, since it might be easy for him to make sure that others are available should he need assistance.

Help Your Parent Participate in New Activities and Make New Friends

If your parent has been too busy over the years with work and family obligations to maintain close friendships and interesting activities, then it's time for some new experiences. Everyone can find something they can do that interests them—as my mother used to say on days when I bugged her one time too many because I was bored.

Help Your Parent Participate in Group Activities

If your parent is a joiner, focus on group activities. Look for a senior center in your area. Often the YMCA (ymca.net) and YWCA (ywca.org) sponsor such activities, as does the National Park Service (NPS.gov). You might also look for activities at your neighborhood community center. I used to live in a planned community with a community center, and in addition to other activities that center offered senior-related exercise and craft classes.

Help Your Parent Participate in Solo Activities
If your parent prefers solo activities, there are reading groups he can follow online, while he keeps up with the latest fiction on his own. He can read this month's book selection, for example, then check in to the Barnes and Noble website, or the GoodReads. com website, and see what the other readers thought of the author's work. If he would prefer an in-person experience, then your parent could attend a reading by an author, whose book he enjoyed, and get an autographed copy of the book. There are also lectures at the local colleges and play subscriptions to local theatres. All of these activities can be enjoyed solo, but they also offer possibilities for social interaction if and when your parent wants it.

Help Your Parent Participate in Volunteer Work (If Possible)
It's sometimes hard to go from a full-time, forty-hour a week plus job (inside or outside of the home) to a zero-hours per week existence. Think outside the box for things that may seem like work to some, but may be much more than a job to your parent. There are volunteer opportunities out there. Maybe being a docent where your parent has to memorize scores of factual details is too much, but there are many other opportunities, such as:

- At the animal shelter, helping clean cages and care for dogs and cats

- At the local vet's, holding the pets while they receive their distemper shots or exams so that they're not as frightened and also so that they start getting more at ease around people, which is often the key to their being adopted and finding a new family

- At the local elementary, talking to the kids about the things your parent knows (planes, or trains, or automobiles, or culinary arts, or farms, or fashion [yes, kids love color, design, and styles, just like you and me], or skyscrapers, or boats, or the law, or medicine, or computers, or engineering, or simply life and growing up when he did—which is a history class for them); if your parent forgets a fact or two, kids, especially kindergarten to second graders, can be especially forgiving of someone who doesn't know the exact right word

Use your imagination and get your parent excited about life again. Life should be fun for him and for you.

As mentioned above, remember your parent's abilities when you suggest activities. Just as you would be careful to place a child in the appropriately-aged play group—and you wouldn't put a seven-year old in a sports group for twelve-year old's—keep that in mind with your parent. If your parent is experiencing a slight mental deficit, make sure that the activity is appropriate and that any needed accommodation is possible and has been arranged.

Keep Emergency Contact Information with Your Parent at All Times

Whether your parent has a cell phone or a special calling device or not, he should have emergency contact information on his person at all times. Your parent's purse or wallet should contain a picture of you, as well as your phone number and address. Hospital, police, and fire and rescue personnel will always review purse and wallet identification information if the person they are with cannot communicate well on his or her own. Make sure this information is clear and easily accessible should the occasion arise that someone has to access it.

More Ideas

If your parent used to read to occupy his time, and now the book is too heavy to hold and the words are too small to read, there are solutions. Go to the library and get your parent large-print books. Find a stand to hold your parent's books. Invest in an inexpensive audiobook service, like Amazon.com's Audible (www.audible.com), for example, so that your parent can listen to his favorite books. Buy him a light weight tablet and connect it to a TV or computer monitor so that your parent can read them right there—on the TV or computer screen.

If your parent uses a computer, see whether it already has software or can accommodate software that takes dictation. That way, even if his hands are too shaky, your parent can write letters to a grandchild or write out a list of things he or she wants you to take care of. Also, encourage your parent to continue with bridge, monopoly, or any other games he has played regularly, so that he does not lose the capacity to do so any sooner than necessary. The more capable your parent feels, the less he will need strangers to take up the slack in his or her life (which will keep him safer and his possessions more secure).

TIP 9

Help Your Parent Maintain Religious Practice

How to Keep Up Your Parent's Faith for Now and for Later

Make sure your church, synagogue, temple, or other house of worship knows that your parent is ill. Not only should your parent's religious practices be continued while he is ill—which sometimes can be done at home—but also, in order to be buried or hold a funeral or memorial service, maintaining his status in his faith may be necessary. In certain faiths, your parent may be required to be a current member in good standing. Though there are faiths that will allow you to come and go as you need to and still allow you to have the necessary marriage, birth, and funeral services, do not count on that kind of latitude. You must find out what the requirements, and possibilities, are for your parent's particular faith. Follow them and make sure that religious officials *know* you are following them.

Do not assume that because a religious official should be able to see that your parent has been ill, that they actually *will* see it and note that fact, or that they will excuse him from some of his religious obligations. They may not. Also, do not assume that understandings and arrangements made with one priest, minister, rabbi, or other official will automatically be honored by another. This can and will affect any services you wish to hold, from availability of the facility, willingness of a minister or priest to perform a service, or even just receiving a bad attitude on the day of the funeral or memorial, which will already be a really bad day.

Provide Access to Religious Services--Either in Person or By Using Technology

In Person

Find out what your parent's faith requires. He may be required to be up-to-date in his attendance, tithing, or in other ways. Often this means that someone needs to be taking him to services, if possible, given your parent's condition and the availability of a qualified person or persons to assist with him. If taking him is not feasible, then someone needs to make the arrangements necessary for religious services to be received at home. Sometimes religious officiants or the church workers who assist them, will visit sick members of the congregation at home to deliver not only appropriate services, but also words of comfort and encouragement. Call, or preferably visit, and find out what's possible for your parent.

Using Technology

Your parent can access his religious services using the Internet, via YouTube for example, or by searching for specific religious leaders or a specific faith. Also, try religious programming on regular TV, cable TV, or programs available through such services as Netflix. There are many religious TV channel service providers now, serving all of the major religions practiced in the world: Christian, Roman Catholic, Episcopalian, Lutheran, Methodist, African Methodist Episcopal, Presbyterian, Baptist, as well as Islamism, Buddhism, Judaism, Hinduism, and Sikhism; you name it. If you own a streaming media player, such as Roku (Roku.com)—where almost 30 different channels displayed when I searched "Christian," Apple TV, or another technology or device, then you will have even more of a selection. Your parent can watch mass from Wisconsin or from the Vatican, watch Joel Osteen even when his show isn't on, watch sermons from T.D. Jakes, or listen to his favorites from Hillsong Church's Hillsong Channel. There are many shows that can soothe, enrich, and enliven your parent's life. Please make use of them.

Help Your Parent Rest in Peace

You want your parent to rest in peace. Key to that is having a right relationship with God and his faith on that final day of his life. You don't know exactly when that day is going to come. So, help your parent continue or start his religious practices, so that he will be helped and comforted, and you will know your parent will be okay where he is going.

How to Maintain Your Parent's Financial Life

- Maintain Your Parent's Bank Accounts

- Get Your Parent a Safe Deposit Box

- Protect Your Parent from Fraud

- Get Your Parent Life Insurance

- Make Sure Your Parent Designates a Power of Attorney

TIP 10

Maintain Your Parent's Bank Accounts

How to Deal with Banking Issues

Get Your Parent an ATM Card (for Checking and Savings Accounts)

Make sure that your parent has an ATM card for all of his bank accounts. (Some people have them for checking but not for savings.) This will help to a great extent. You—or anyone with your parent—can go and withdraw funds up to a certain limit, without needing your parent there to walk in, without needing his signature on anything, and without needing to hassle with a line inside the bank.

When your parent can no longer drive himself, someone else dictates where he lives—or his food, medicine, and schedule—retaining his ability to withdraw twenty dollars from his own bank account can be very important. It maintains your parent's dignity and sense of autonomy. Age or infirmity do not alter our desire to be who we are. All of us feel pretty much the way we always have felt about ourselves. We see ourselves as viable people and want to be treated that way by others. You don't suddenly look in the bathroom mirror and say, "Well, I'm old now, so I guess I'll just let people boss me around and enjoy it." It doesn't happen that way. Autonomy, the sense that we are individuals who have a say-so in our own lives, remains important throughout life. For many of us, it is something we only miss when it is challenged. Try to give your parent enough leeway to retain at least some of this very important feeling of autonomy. Let your parent stay who he is for as long as you can.

Find an Alternative to Signing His or Her Name—Such as a Power of Attorney

There are times, however, when an ATM card will not do the trick. These are times when your parent will have to walk into the bank, talk to a teller, and sign his name. Maybe it will be just a matter of record keeping. Let's say the bank has changed hands, is updating its ATM cards, and wants each customer to update his photo and back of card signature the next time he visits the bank (and, yes, this happened to my mom and I). Perhaps your parent has direct withdrawals from his checking or savings account and the amount is too high; it needs to be updated to prevent overages. Maybe your parent still has bonds or certificates of deposit (CDs) that he has been holding on to and needs to cash them in. None of these transactions can be handled using an ATM card. Granted, these are not everyday situations or transactions. Nonetheless, they occur. When they do, it's usually a surprise, and you usually need a solution, fast. Try to anticipate these odd kinds of needs and have a way to handle them. To do so, your parent needs an alternative to walking into the bank, talking to a teller, and signing his name. That means that either his presence and ID will have to suffice and a bank manager will approve his transactions, or a designated person (the person he has named in his power of attorney), probably you, will need to be allowed to sign for him. Make sure your parent's bank will allow at least one of these types of transactions. Sometimes, this process simply requires that you fill out a form and have it notarized. (We had to go through such a process with a notary for my mom.) Find out what the process is for your parent and do it now, before you need it. By the way, if you do get this permission, try getting it in writing or at least get the name and title of the person who gave it to you and keep it handy for future reference.

Become a Signatory on Your Parent's Accounts

Consider becoming a signatory on your parent's bank account. Why? Because not only will the circumstances described earlier in this tip occur at some point, but also at some point your parent may no longer be able to reason about his banking affairs, and he will need you to be able to handle these issues for him.

If both parents are still living, and if the parent with Alzheimer's or other dementia has a joint bank account, then the other parent can definitely decide on issues and sign, because the money belongs to both parties. If the money is in an individual account and your parents are married, it may take some time, but the other parent can probably still access the funds once ID, medical statements from doctors, etc. are exchanged with the bank. If, however, this is your only living parent, and your name is not on the account, then that money isn't going anywhere until the will is read, or probate occurs, or some other legal procedure is endured. This is money that cannot be used to pay the mortgage on the house. If you've taken time off from work to care for your parent and your income has been greatly reduced, this may be money you need to feed your parent. The bank will not just give you access to the funds. So, consider what your situation is and how comfortable you and your parent feel with your name being on his account. As I mention in the tip on powers of attorney (POA), the POA is not always a magic bullet in these situations, and banks and other offices do not automatically allow you access to accounts just because you have one, but it is a start. You can always talk to your parent's attorney about any problems you encounter and also about any appropriate alternatives to the POA in order to expedite handling your parent's financial affairs (such as setting up a guardianship, trust, or representative payee, if any of these are appropriate). Consider these points carefully.

TIP 11

Get Your Parent a Safe Deposit Box

How to Deal with Safe Deposit Boxes

Help your parent get a safe deposit box and use it. Fill it with all of your parent's banking information, information on all bills and debts, a copy of your parent's will and power of attorney, detailed notes and stipulations about funeral arrangements, family history, select jewelry, private papers, or other cherished items.

Keep Track of the Safe Deposit Box Number and Keys

Your parent might have gotten that safe deposit box ten or fifteen years ago, thinking it would save you kids some time. Now, no one knows where the key is. That's a bit of a problem. It's not one that can't be surmounted, but it is one that will require two IDs and some cash. Don't blame the bank—though you're allowed a few curse words here. It's better for the bank to be suspicious than not. You do not want the bank saying, "Hey, come in and take whatever you want," do you? Well, that's the alternative. The moral of the story is, keep the safe deposit box key somewhere safe and yet easy to access. Make sure that your siblings or at least two other people know its location. (Siblings, you know who among you is the most trustworthy and the most organized. Choose that person to hold the key and ward off the others.) Without the key, as I mentioned, if you want to access the box, even after you've spent your three trips convincing the bank to talk to you, they are going to charge you about $200 to drill the box open. When you go to the bank, bring your power of attorney (POA), death certificate (if appropriate), photo ID, and cash or credit to pay the fee.

If your parent has not already secured a safe deposit box, go with him. You need to make sure the bank knows who you are, and if possible, you need to get in writing that you have your parent's permission to access the box. You also need to know what your parent is storing in the box, its importance or significance, and how urgent it will be for you to access the box contents upon your parent's death. For example, the box could contain an updated will or financial documents that will help to defer immediate expenses, or it could contain drawings you did when you were three. Both are good. One is urgent; the other can wait.

Keep Track of the Bank Where the Safe Deposit Box Is Located

Banks are bought and sold. Banks move from one building to another. So, keep tabs on the bank where your parent has his safe deposit box. Do not depend on the bank to notify you of these changes. Keep abreast of the situation. You need to know that the bank hasn't been sold to another bank and that it still exists (or at least what the new name and new location of the bank is). You need to know that the box fees are being faithfully paid so that the contents of the box will be there when needed. Otherwise, the bank will take the contents of the box and either keep them or toss them out. So once again, you, my friend, are going to be out of luck and probably banging your head against a very hard wall if you don't pay attention and you let this happen. Therefore, don't.

Put Valuables in a Safe Deposit Box

Safe deposit boxes are a great place to store valuables away from home. Review your agreement with the bank that houses your safe deposit box to learn what items are appropriate to include in yours. If a larger box is required to house the items you wish to store, see one of the bank's representatives to secure that change.

In a safe deposit box, your parent's valuables can be protected from home fire and flood disasters. They also can be protected from family members or others who might remove objects without permission. Remember, when people are ill, they have various visitors—from neighbors, to visiting strangers, to distant relatives, to service workers of all kinds—who have access to their valuables. When people are concerned about losing someone, they can do stupid things. These visitors will be in your parent's home at a time when no one may be paying attention to what they are doing since your parent's health and care will be everyone's main focus. You should of course be careful about who is allowed into your parent's home, but more importantly you should take precautions. Protect people from themselves and protect your parent by removing valuable items. By valuables I mean both the kind that cost a lot of money and the ones that have no marketable value but mean a lot to you and are irreplaceable. Once your parent's valuables are in the safe deposit box, they can be retrieved by someone with the family's authority. That person can then either return the items to the family home at an appropriate time or distribute them per your parent's will or per other arrangements.

Use Caution When Putting Certain Items in a Safe Deposit Box

Your parent should consider carefully whether he wants to place private papers such as journals or diaries in a safe deposit box. If he does, he should not make it obvious that these are the objects he is storing. Unfortunately, banks have nosy and unethical people, just like any other place. This is not the place to store information about his long-lost love child (if he has one), his Swiss bank account, or other information meant for only one or two people in the world. He needs to tell the people who need to know that kind of information, preferably early and privately. Then, when he is gone, they can handle the information at an appropriate time and in an appropriate manner without the prying eyes of others.

TIP 12

Protect Your Parent from Fraud

How to Lower the Possibility of Fraud

Sometimes dementia, along with loneliness, frustration, and simply being a kind and trusting person, can be a problem when mixed with untrustworthy or unsavory groups or individuals. After coming home from work one day and finding a representative from a questionable political group standing in our living room demanding a check from my mom, I learned to watch for any signs that she was being taken advantage of, either in person or electronically (which seems to be a popular method these days).

Notice Unusual Behavior

- Is your parent beginning to give money to too many organizations?

- Have the people visiting your parent changed?

- Do you find your parent being open to religious, political, or social groups that are unusual for him?

- Are you concerned that some of the people surrounding your parent now may not be legitimate or in his best interest? Quite simply, are you concerned that these individuals may not be on the up and up and may be taking advantage of your parent?

- Is your parent buying too many lottery tickets all of a sudden or is he believing every letter or e-mail that says he has won millions in a contest or lottery that he never entered?

Monitor Your Parent

What I'm getting at here is that especially if fraud is a concern, you need to begin monitoring your parent's affairs—his e-mail, letters, bank accounts, etc. You need to see what's going on before there is a problem. Here is my word to the wise, however, please do it in a way that does not bully your parent. (See Tip 6, I discuss some technologies that could assist you in monitoring your parent's online activity.)

Monitoring is to help your parent, not hurt him, and it should be done with tact, kindness, and consideration—and with permission if at all possible. If it is a matter of your parent's safety, sometimes niceties have to suffer. Take care of your parent's safety needs first and foremost. But try to maintain his sense of dignity while you help him. Your parent is still an adult. You don't really have the right to run roughshod over him. You have a duty to care for him. So, remember, let your words and actions taste more like honey than vinegar to your parent, and perhaps he will allow you to help him help himself.

Handle Unusual or Unwelcome Letters or E-mails If They Start Showing Up in Your Parent's Mailbox

If unusual or unwelcome letters or e-mails start showing up in your parent's mailbox, do not think you are being overprotective if you want to begin to monitor his e-mail or letters, or to review these exchanges. It will protect your parent and give you peace of mind. Try these suggestions:

- Suggest that you can help your parent with his technology. Do not grab the keyboard out of your parent's hands and insist he do things your way.

- Offer to sit with your parent and review the letters or e-mail messages that come in for him. Do not just delete messages or throw out letters because you think they are unimportant or a waste of time.

- Call your parent's bank if you notice questionable letters or e-mails demanding or promising funds. Better yet, set up a bank account that you can monitor online.

Handle Unusual or Unwelcome People If They Start Showing Up on Your Parent's Doorstep

If unusual or unwelcome people start showing up on your parent's doorstep, alert a neighbor, that is if he still lives in the kind of neighborhood where people have known each other and each others' children for most of their lives. If you do not have that situation, you may be putting your parent in more danger by alerting a stranger to his vulnerabilities. In this case, instead of alerting people with no need to know and no legitimate and strong connection to your parent, install an outside camera so that all visitors are on-screen at all times. If they are legitimate, it will not matter to them. If they are not, you may be saving your parent and yourself time, money, security, or life itself. I do not say these things to frighten you unnecessarily. I say these things because, as they say, the world is not what it used to be. Even in those "good old days," sometimes people took advantage of others they saw as weaker or less savvy than themselves. Why? Just because. If I knew the answer to that, I could rule the world. Therefore, remember what P. T. Barnum said about a fool being born every minute, and be savvy enough to avoid playing that role.

Also, consider ways to decrease your parent's need for these new people. The dementia may have your parent feeling isolated and lonely, making any warm-sounding person a plus. He needs other things and people to look forward to seeing and engaging. Give this to him. Read the tip "Help Your Parent Maintain Social Contacts."

TIP 13

Get Insurance for Your Parent to Help Him Protect His Family and to Provide Funds to Pay Off Final Expenses

How to Help Your Parent Provide for Others After He's Gone through Insurance

Your parent needs life insurance. He needs it if he has a spouse who has counted on his salary as part of his or her own financial survival. He needs it if he has children, especially minor children, who will need to be provided for in the future. He also needs it if he has a house—and people who will still need to reside in that house—and that house has a mortgage that may be difficult to manage on one salary. Your parent probably neither wants to leave his children broke, nor his spouse struggling to make the mortgage payments or having to move out of the house he or she has come to call home. Your parent might also need to have a policy to cover outstanding debts, like the loan Uncle David gave him or to cover or help with the final expense of a funeral or memorial service.

This discussion is going to be very general, because I am not a life insurance expert, but it should get you started thinking about what you need to do to secure your parent's and your future. *Remember, it will take time after your parent's passing to redeem any insurance policy, and you may need other money to pay for services, and so forth, up front, but it will be worth it in the end.*

If your parent has no one depending on him, then perhaps other options will suffice. For example, if your parent does not have life insurance, but no mortgage or other major or monthly payments will need to be made after his death, then perhaps only a small final expense policy needs to be purchased so that funeral and other final expenses can be paid promptly. Or, perhaps your parent could simply start socking away the equivalent of an insurance premium each month to cover those costs. If you do purchase an insurance policy, however, be careful to make sure that the policy your parent gets is worth it.

Learn about Accidental Death and Dismemberment Insurance Policies

An accidental death and dismemberment policy could be helpful if your parent were to die as the result of an accident or if he were to live, but had been dismembered due to an accident. Sometimes people assume that the situation is going to be their passing away and someone receiving their life insurance. If someone does not pass away, however, he may not have adequate insurance, insurance that will cover himself (in the case of your parent) or the insurance that will cover himself and those dependent on him (in the case of your parent with dependents.

I discuss how these policies can also be carried by you to assist your parent in one of the sections that follow.

One point about accidental death and dismemberment policies, however, they are good only if that happens to be the way your parent (or you) die or are injured. These policies may not have any value if your parent or you die in bed of an illness (unless that illness is somehow related to the concepts of accidental death or dismemberment). Therefore, get these policies if you want and if the circumstances suggesting them are appropriate, but please also consider the many policies that will pay out in the usual situations that happen to most people—such as death after a long or short illness. These could prove far more appropriate for your parent to have. Read on.

Learn about Life Insurance Policies

Your parent is most likely going to die of causes related to some illness or condition, either at his home, your home, or in a nursing home. When that happens, there should be a regular life insurance policy in place, one that will pay enough to cover burial expenses (including money for a wake, meal, or whatever other activities are appropriate for your family and its traditions), money to pay off credit cards, remaining medical bills, and if possible any other debt your parent has incurred. If it is not possible to cover all of these things, ask an attorney whether it is better to focus on the burial and deal with the other issues later or alter your expected funeral services and put funds toward resolving the debt. It will depend for the most part on whether the estate will have to pay for the remaining debt by selling your parent's home or other assets. If this is the house you grew up in, still live in, or for another reason want to keep, be frank with your attorney about what your goals are so that you can make sure that your parent gets and keeps the insurance (read "future security") *that you will need once he is gone*. Once these items are covered, you will be able to focus on your parent—and on all the little issues swirling around him—with some peace of mind.

Consider Adding to Your Parent's Current Insurance
Peace of Mind for Cents a Week

Check to see whether your parent already has one of those policies that will pay an appropriate amount, let's say $10,000, $20,000, or $30,000, to cover final expenses. If he does, that's great. If not, consider getting one. The idea of thinking about funeral expenses may not seem like a pleasant one, but it is better now than later, when you are wondering how to afford a simple burial for your parent. Ask your insurance agent. Watch for TV commercials. Ask your friends. You can find a policy that is both affordable and worth the small but still additional expense.

Consider Adding to Your Own Current Insurance
Cover Yourself Just in Case (Especially If You Are Your Parent's Only Financial Support)

Get your own insurance policy and designate your parent as the beneficiary, just in case. If you are the sole support of your parent, if you are paying for part or all of your parent's care, what happens if you have an accident and someone has to take care of you? How will your parent manage then? It happens, so please consider the possibility as you are making your plans. If you would have an Accidental Death and Dismemberment insurance policy to cover your spouse and dependent children, then please consider having a policy that will cover your dependent parent in those same circumstances (and consider the parents on both sides of the family—even if they are not now ill—if those relationships make it an appropriate thing to do). If you tell the insurance agent that you have a dependent parent who will need to be covered by any insurance you have, he or she will be able to recommend appropriate policies.

I carried both an accidental death and dismemberment policy and a life insurance policy while my mother lived. If anything had happened to me, at least one of these policies would have been available to pay the mortgage on her home, and her debt (as well as my own debt) in part if I had an accident but survived, in full upon my death. My insurance also would have paid for her stay in a good-quality nursing facility until her death. I found it helped me sleep at night. Her future wasn't dependent on anybody picking up the slack after I was gone. I was assured the money would be there for her to be okay, even if the next person to handle the power of attorney needed to access the funds for other items.

Understand Insurance Payouts and Timing

It's Helpful Money, Not Instant Money

Please note one thing: getting the life insurance company to pay out on your parent's policy is going to require having the contact information for the agent, the policy number(s), and time. If you don't have this information close at hand, try the Lost Policy Locator Service on the National Association of Insurance Commissioners' (NAIC) website (https://eapps.naic.org/life-policy-locator/#/welcome). Do not expect to receive a check the week after your parent passes away or in time for the deposit on the funeral service. Most likely, the money from the policy will arrive later, in time to reimburse whoever lays out the cash or credit for the services. It probably will not, however, be there in time to pay for the services up front, and many funeral homes and churches expect to be paid up front. (And yes, you do often have to pay something for the use of a church, even if it's just to pay the pastor for his time.) Having said that, life insurance is usually guaranteed money, in the sense that a policy for $50,000—remember this is true if and only if the policy is fully paid up per whatever agreement you sign—should and probably will pay out $50,000 after identification and request procedures have been fulfilled. Consider getting a life insurance policy.

(**Note**: I realize the amount above may seem high. I am using it to say that **if you can replace at least a portion of the deceased person's income—salary or retirement funds—for one year, that could make a huge difference for you and your family**. Therefore, please consider more insurance *if it is affordable for you*. Do not ruin your finances now to do it, but also *do not forget what life, and your finances, will be like without the other person around to contribute*. Life insurance is not just to pay for the funeral or memorial, it is also to help you and your family get on with your lives, to live with a roof over your heads, sufficient food, etc. while you sort out things without your parent there. Maybe this is not an issue for you, your siblings, or his or her surviving spouse if there is one, but then again maybe it is. Realistically assess your individual situation.)

My Story

I wanted to add that insurance companies were the best institutions with which I dealt while handling my mother's estate. The money was the exact amount expected. There were no arguments, no aggravation, just prompt, efficient service. They had an ID verification process that was sufficient enough to make me feel safe and secure that any funds my mother entrusted to them were well handled, but not more arduous than it needed to be. I dealt with a few companies and had a similar experience at each one. Two companies, American General® and Met Life®, standout in the professional and efficient manner in which they treated me. This may not sound like something spectacular, but in the world of estates and bureaucracies from which I have only recently gained my freedom, it was almost unbelievable. In the future, I would definitely use an insurance policy myself to help secure my loved ones' futures knowing these companies (from what I have seen so far) will be true to their words.

Last Words – Good People, the Ultimate Insurance

Insurance policies can be expensive. Remember one thing, whether you can afford and obtain insurance policies or not, your best insurance is always people around your parent who care. If these suggestions seem or are prohibitive or just won't work for any reason, then consider the insurance of human relationships. Who do you know and trust who can look in on your parent, take meals to your parent, sit with your parent, or make sure that the right people are called and the right forms are filled out to get your parent into an appropriate facility or location where he can be cared for? It doesn't have to be the same person for each activity. Answer those questions and that may be the best insurance policy of all. Keep friends and family around your parent and keep friends and family around yourself, and both of you will always be comforted.

TIP 14

Setup a Power of Attorney to Ensure Your Parent's Future Medical (Health care) and Financial Well-Being

How to Make Sure Your Parent Has a Power of Attorney (POA)

Caveat (Warning)
am not an attorney. The information in this tip is general and intended to get you thinking prior to your seeing an attorney for advice. Do not rely on this information as a substitute for the professional advice of and direct contact with an attorney.

Ask Whether There's a Power of Attorney (POA) and Locate the Paperwork, or Setup a New POA
Your parent needs to decide who will take care of his money and who will have the right to make medical decisions on his behalf while he is still living. Those things are achieved through the use of a power of attorney (POA). The power of attorney will let everyone know who has been designated to have the right to access bank accounts to care for your parent. It will also tell everyone who is in charge of your parent's health care decision making should he become incapacitated. Make sure your parent has the best chance of continuing to live life as he sees fit by making sure he puts these decisions down in writing.

Find out whether or not your parent has designated someone to have POA. Usually, the attorney that draws up the will would be the same person to handle the

POA. Thus, this paper may be with your parent's will. Ask your parent. If they don't know where it is, contact your parent's lawyer, the other parent, your parent's best friend, or a close neighbor, and don't forget to search drawers.

If there is still no sign of a POA, and they have an attorney in their lives, consider going to him to draw up the POA. If there is no attorney to contact, then consider starting your search for an attorney on your computer. You can access FindLaw.com and search under "Elder Care Attorney" to find and select someone appropriate. You can also use a friend's recommendation, or respond to a lawyer's advertisement.

You may not think a POA is important, but it comes in handy when your parent has a $500 copay on a prescription, you do not have the $500 to give him, and he has $500 in the bank, however, the money is in an account that he cannot access—because he doesn't have an ATM card and the bank won't allow a withdrawal because he cannot sign his name to the withdrawal form. (I've been there.)

Understand Issues with Using a Power of Attorney (POA)

Beware that the POA is not a slam dunk. Sometimes, in some places, you may still experience problems. After the incident described above, my mom and I decided to alert other banking institutions so that we could avoid having that problem again in the future. So as soon as we could, we went to a different bank, one where we both had accounts and one we both visited frequently. I presented the POA and asked that they put it on file there to make it clear what the situation was with my parent. I was told that it wouldn't be easy to achieve that goal, that is, to gain access to my mother's banking, with just that piece of paper and my ID, even with my mom standing there with me. A very nice and very savvy banker made a suggestion, however, he suggested that my mom add me to her accounts. That day, she did just that, and I will always be grateful to that banker. It has saved me many times. This act made my mom's bank accounts Joint Bank Accounts, with me as the other signatory on the account.

In numerous situations in which I was not on an account and offered my POA— often with my mother present and consenting and with me offering more than one ID—I was denied access to whatever resource I requested and usually had to wage a campaign to gain access. Sometimes, I even had to garner the assistance of her attorney. Not that I minded taking days off work to drive into the city for an hour, finding and paying for parking, walking my mother arm-in-arm three blocks to the credit union (because I could not leave her standing alone by herself while I parked), and then being told that my mother, who banked at this credit union for over thirty years, would not be allowed to access her own money because she could no longer sign her name to the proper form. These are the kinds of things that are going to happen to you regularly. It took three trips, on three separate days, to get access to my mom's credit union account. If you count the vacation time I used and the years off my life that they subtracted by the sheer aggravation they caused me, it was a pretty costly task. Save yourself the frustration, and have your parent add you to his accounts *now*, while everyone is smiling and willing to give you, as a new customer, good customer service. Do not wait until you are begging and wondering why they will not honor your POA and help. They may be trying to figure out whether you are sincere or simply trying to keep your elderly parent's money. It happens. Yes, banks are cautious for a reason, but that will not matter to you after you've wasted a day on one of these errands. Protect your parent, but also protect your health, sanity, and future wages. Get your name somewhere on the account, have a picture ID on file, and if you can, visit frequently with your parent so that the bank knows who you are.

Learn About Alternatives to the Power of Attorney (POA)

Because of the issues that I had with a POA, which I discussed above, you might want to ask your attorney whether there is an alternative to the POA. As mentioned above, you can become a signatory on your parent's account, making the account a joint account that you both hold. There are other alternatives out there—perhaps some kind of **trust** or designating someone as a **representative payee**, but you can only be sure of any of these alternatives by asking a qualified attorney, and I am not one. If your parent does not have an attorney, then use some of the resources listed in the "Wills," tip in this book, such as FindLaw.com or National Academy of Elder Law Attorneys (http://www.naela.org/), for more information on finding an attorney. Also give a read to information such as Virginia's Division for the Aging website, under Alternatives to Guardianship, (www.vda.virginia.gov), which discusses POAs, trusts, and representative payees and which may give you the information you need to start this conversation with your parent and your own attorney, in your state. Regardless of the sources you read or consider, remember to always see an attorney. Only an attorney can give you the proper advice to protect your parent.

How To Know When It's Time For More Care And What To Do

- Help Your Parent Put Down the Car Keys (When Appropriate)

  - Transportation and Driving

  - Putting Away Your Parent's Car Keys and Making Other Arrangements

- Assess Your Parent's Need for More Advanced Care

- Care and Housing / Living Situation Options

  - Staying in His Own Home

  - Moving in with You

  - Moving in with Someone Else

  - Moving into a Facility

TIP 15

When It's Time, Don't Be Afraid to Take Your Parent's Car Keys

How to Start Paying Attention to Your Parent's Driving

I don't like the title I chose for this section, but I felt I had to choose it. I don't like saying this. I wish there were a day when each of us would know our limitations automatically and could adjust accordingly. We'd just set down our car keys and say, "Okay, I'm ready for something else." Sometimes that's the case, and everything goes well. We just don't drive anymore; we get rides. Other times, we think we can make just one more trip and it doesn't work out. Or we don't even consider whether we can make one more trip because we are unaware of a new limitation that has fallen on us. Therefore, sometimes we need help from our families and friends to put down the car keys, when it's time. As I related earlier in this book, see Tip 1, I took them—my mom's car keys—after she had trouble finding her way home from a location she had regularly visited, on a path she had traveled many times and knew by heart. I did it as subtly and as nicely as I could. Months later, I learned that she suffered from multi-infarct (or vascular) dementia.

What follows is a strong warning. I give it because often we miss that first odd event or we discount its importance. Someone who looks like they are drunk or have the flu may be experiencing something entirely different. Remember the scene with Steve's mother in the first Sex and the City movie?[18] That's what I'm talking about. *If you suspect your parent may have had a stroke or other serious occurrence that created his behavior, or you have any concerns that he needs immediate care, take him to the*

---

18 "Sex and the City," 2008 film, Michael Patrick King, writer and director, based on a book by Candace Bushnell, IMDb.com, accessed November 21, 2017, http://www.imdb.com/title/tt1000774/?ref_=fn_al_tt_2

emergency room now, immediately. That care could make a major, long-term differ-
ence in your parent's prognosis. His future health could depend on those first hours.

Have the "Stop Driving" Talk, If Necessary

Some people are fans of honesty. I am usually one of them, except when it comes to taking your parent's keys.

If you have a parent who can handle the "You shouldn't drive anymore" conversation, then by all means have that conversation. Have it early. Have it frequently, if necessary, and agree to a process or procedure when you, or another person deemed responsible for the determination, can say, "It's time to stop driving," and your parent will heed that determination and indeed stop.

If your parent insists he is fine, despite driving over curves or getting lost or disoriented on the road, then I am personally—for myself and those dear to me—a fan of doing whatever you have to do to keep your parent off the road. If you cannot bring yourself to do it overtly, tell him you lost the car keys, and offer to drive your parent wherever he needs to go. (Always make sure your parent has transportation in case of an emergency.)

Remember, it may be too late once your parent's car has jumped the curve and hit or mowed down innocent people who were out for a stroll. The tragedy will have already happened. It also may be too late when your parent is lost on the road at nine o'clock at night, no one knows where he is, and your parent cannot figure out where he is himself, or how to contact you, or how to find anyone to help him. Start those conversations with your parent, and if you already have had similar upsetting situations with him about the car, please take his keys, at least temporarily, and get your parent to a doctor. Do it as kindly and respectfully as possible, but save your stomach lining and possibly his and other peoples' lives by doing it!

Before you apply what I have said to your situation, please be clear about what I actually am saying and what I am not saying. Here is a list of what I am *not* saying:

- *I am __not saying__,* "Wow, mom got lost trying to find that new store, so take her keys."

- *I am __not__ saying,* "Anyone over the age of <u>fill in the blank</u> should be prevented from driving."

- **I am _not_ saying**, "Take the keys of any older person having health problems."

I am saying that if there were no other issues and everything was the same as it usually is for your parent, and he could not make a successful car trip, that is a significant warning sign to you. I am saying that if someone is driving to or from a place that he has driven to and from repeatedly and successfully many times, and he suddenly cannot complete the trip, then there is a problem, and taking his keys might be the first step to solving it. I am saying that you need to heed the warning. What do I mean by "heed the warning"? I mean take your parent to the doctor and find out what's going on. Maybe it will be an inner ear infection that threw off his balance, or medication that affected his reasoning and perception skills. Maybe for your parent it really was just the new buildings, and when the two of you went back to the same location—with him driving—he was able to drive the car just fine. Or maybe it is a major problem. Regardless, you need to take the keys and get your parent to a doctor.

Know When to Call in the Doctor

It Might Not Be Alzheimer's or Dementia; It Could Be Something Else; See a Doctor

Don't just jump to the conclusion that the problem is dementia of some kind. Problems with driving could stem from many things. (Also, don't just assume that he had a bad day that will never repeat itself.)

- **Issues with Eyesight:** Is your parent truly behaving in a demented way, or is he or she having issues that driving glasses or special night-vision eyewear would help or resolve? Does your parent have cataracts? These can affect depth perception and make things like navigating stairs in and out of the house difficult or affect other abilities. If cataracts are the problem, can they be safely removed at this stage of your parent's health?

- **Issues with Your Parent's Car:** Are there problems with the car itself? Are the headlights functioning properly to allow your parent to see the road and street signs well enough? Are interior lights allowing your parent to view driving directions or make a phone call easily when he pulls off the road to reassess his situation? Did your parent really miscalculate the curve or that parking space, or are the tires on his car bald and slipping on the wet pavement? Sometimes elderly parents skimp on things like car maintenance in order to live on a fixed income.

- **Issues with Other Medical Problems:** Has your parent had a complete checkup lately? Does he have any known, ongoing health problems that have been left unattended? Sometimes parents do not understand how to use their health insurance, and they think they cannot get the help they sorely need.

The only way to know is by going to the doctor, having the tests or other procedures, and listening to whatever information your doctor provides.

Until Your Doctor's Appointment

As I've said, until your parent sees the doctor, prevent him from driving. Drive him yourself or have someone you trust drive him.

Provide Alternative Transportation

For many people, transportation is a must. Your parent may still be working (His fitness for work is something else that *might* need to be evaluated if the driving issues prove to be only one problem he is having. Your doctor can help with this assessment). Your parent might need to get food or other supplies. He might have an emergency and need to leave home rapidly. Therefore, you must make sure you or someone else close by can be there and take your parent where he needs to go.

Have an alternative method of transportation for him, and make sure it will work. What do I mean by that? Well, people get lost on bus lines just as they do in traffic. So, a senior transportation bus, where the driver bears some responsibility for your parent, might be a good idea. (Try to get to know the driver and keeps tabs on the bus company.)

Better yet, maybe you can drive him. If you make an outing of driving your parent, taking him to a leisurely lunch and the barber, bank, and dry cleaners, for example, that will go over better than rushing your parent through errands and refusing to take him to the places he needs to go. Your parent has a life. Let him go to the places he frequents and handle the tasks he needs to complete to feel he is living life as he should.

And you know what you might discover? You might discover that you do not just have a parent; you have an interesting companion, a person that in many ways you barely know, a person who just might become a good friend.

Talk About Your Concern That He Will Drive Anyway, If Necessary
If you are afraid your parent will try to drive anyway, then talk to him about your concerns and reinforce the fact that once you see the doctor, the situation will be clearer. Be as cooperative as you can be—because you are talking to another adult, not a child—but the fact that you were nice to your parent will not soothe you if you let him drive and he harms himself or others. So be firm, but be respectful.

After Your Doctor's Appointment
If it's just a case of eye glasses needing adjustment, of cataracts needing removal, of medication needing change, follow the best medical advice you can obtain and handle these matters according your doctor's, your, and your parent best efforts. If it is more, such as Alzheimer's, other dementia, or something else, make sure your doctor discusses driving and whether it can and should still be a part of your parent's life. If it is to remain a part of your parent's life for now, ask for suggestions from the doctor on monitoring the situation. If driving can no longer be a part of your parent's life, consider all of the things you did in this tip before the doctor's appointment, when maintaining both your parent's freedom and his safety were paramount, and incorporate some of those ideas and techniques as part of your daily routine, if your doctor approves of them.

Consider Swapping a State ID for Your Parent's Driver's License, If Necessary
If advanced age and state of health warrant, you may also, depending on your situation, want to talk about obtaining a State ID in place of your parent's driver's license. The State ID is used by people who do not drive, and therefore do not need a license, but do find that they need a form of identification. The State ID contains all of the same type information as a driver's license, but it does not provide permission to drive. When you obtain this State ID—which can be done either during the time you would normally update a driver's license or at any time at your local department of motor vehicle administration—you turn in the driver's license permanently. My mom had one of these State IDs after it was clear that due to her advanced age and condition she would no longer be driving. Because this

is a permanent change, make sure that you *give it plenty of thought before* making this change for your parent. Remember, it will effect his daily life and yours.

Precautions, If No Driving Problems Exist Yet

Assess Your Parent's Driving Regularly

If you haven't had a driving incident with your parent, that's good. I would still suggest, however, that as a precaution you ride along with him occasionally to observe how he is driving. Consider varying the days and times. That way, you can see whether he drives well not only in slower traffic during the week day, but also during rush hour's faster traffic and on the weekend. Make sure you are 100 percent comfortable with what you observe. If not, see your doctor or any specialist he recommends, such as an eye doctor for sight problems or an ear specialist for issues regarding sounds of a siren or other traffic warnings.

Know Where Your Parent Travels

It's also a good idea to make note of where your parent drives, who he visits, what days he travels, and what routes he uses. This kind of information could be useful to you one day, whether your parent is experiencing any driving problems now or not.

Know Where to Find Identifying Information, such as Photographs of Your Parent

As with anyone you love, having a recent photo of your parent on hand is a good idea. Should your parent get lost or should you need proof that you are indeed your parent's child—for example, if your parent cannot recall who you are—a photograph can come in handy. Make sure you have a photo of your parent alone, as well as one of the two of you together. If you just turned for a minute and your parent wandered away while out with you, a photo gives you something to show people on the street who might have seen your father. If you ever have to contact authorities because your parent has gone missing, a photo gives you something to give police to help them with their search for your mother. Furthermore, if necessary, it also gives you something that a TV station can show on screen during their news announcement, which will reach many more people and make finding your parent more likely.

TIP 16

Assess Your Parent's Need for More Advanced Care

How to Think about Your Parent's Condition Now

n this section, I am assuming that your parent can no longer fully function on his own. Your parent's limitations may be minor and remain that way for some time, or your parent's limitations may be severe. Please read on.

Assess What Your Parent's Condition Is Now

Think of your parent in terms of the rooms of a typical house (plus the area just outside it). He needs to be able to function in each of these rooms: living room, dining room, kitchen, laundry, bedroom, bathroom. Where your parent has trouble functioning, he needs either help to do the activities required or for someone else to do these activities for him. If you consider these aspects, you will know what housing/living situation best fits his care needs. (Housing/Living situations are discussed in Tip 18.) The main question should always be: Is he aware enough to handle himself in this area without concern about injury? And if the answer is ever, "I'm not sure" or "No, he cannot do that without me being concerned about injury," then you know you need someone there to help him with that activity in that area. Let your answers to the questions (not mine, yours) and your own concerns indicate what you need to discuss with your doctor and your parent as the three of you decide what is best for your parent now.

What You Need to Consider about Your Parent's Condition
Consider the questions below and add some of your own in order to analyze and come to some conclusions about the status of your parent's condition. (A form with this checklist is available at the end of this tip.):

Living Room

- Can he turn the TV on and off?

- Can he find a specific channel on the TV—whether it's organized or just clicking around the entire dial?

- Can he select a movie or TV show and know what he's watching?

- Can he engage in a conversation? Does he talk or mostly listen?

- Does he still answer the telephone and understand the interaction?

- Does he talk on the telephone to friends?

- Does he have friends that come over to visit or would come over if the housing set up were more favorable?

Dining Room

- Can he sit up and feed himself or does he need help?

- Does he still have the manual dexterity to wield a knife and fork or does he have arthritis or motor-skill problems that prevent him from using his hands well?

- Does he have trouble chewing any foods? Does he need dental work to assist with this?

- Does he need anyone to cut up his food into small pieces or to prepare soups or other more liquid-type nourishment?

Kitchen

- Can he prepare meals for himself? Are these just small meals, a re-heated dinner from the night before, or actually cooking from scratch?

- Can he still use the microwave, toaster oven, kitchen grill, or stove?

- Can he purchase groceries at the store, or must someone else drive him, or go there in his place?

- Can he prepare any special foods or dietary supplements that his doctor has ordered?

- Can he wash the dishes, either at the sink or in a dishwasher?

Laundry

- Can he organize, wash, and dry the laundry, keeping the clothes in good order?

Bedroom

- Does he still walk (ambulatory) or is he in a wheelchair?

- Does he need help in and out of bed?

- Does he need assistance due to incontinence issues (more frequent changing of your parent's bedding and clothing, an increased need for bathing or washing up, etc.)?

- Is he easily frightened and needs someone by his bedside?

- Does he have a tendency to wander around and needs someone to always keep an eye on his whereabouts?

- Does he need someone by his bedside to assure administration of medication or other treatments?

Bathroom

- Can your parent get into and out of the bath tub or shower?

- Does he still understand a hot water vs. cold water tap?

- Does he still understand when the water in the tub is too high, or that the surface of the tub or floor could be slippery?

- Will someone need to help him bathe, either by securing him in place in the tub, or actually cleaning him?

- Does he need to be lifted or carried there?

- Does he need assistance using the toilet?

Outside

- Does your parent need assistance to go outside for some sunshine?

- Does he need someone to assist with pushing a wheelchair? If so, does he need an electric model or simply assistance?

- Can he walk on sidewalks, grass, or gravel without easily falling?

- Can he go for walks down the block and back alone or is there a danger that he might wander and go missing?

- Can he still participate in any outdoor activities (jogging, walking the dog around the block) without getting lost or disoriented?

The questions above have been put in a form, the Assess Your Parent's Condition Checklist, which follows. Use the form to note your parent's abilities. Review it before your parent's next doctor's visit or consider taking it along with you for the doctor to review, so that he or she fully understands your parent's situation.

Checklist

ASSESS YOUR PARENT'S CONDITION CHECKLIST (Circle Your Response)

Living Room

Can he turn the TV on and off?   **Yes / No**

Can he find a specific channel on the TV—
whether it's organized or just clicking around
the entire dial?   **Yes / No**

Can he select a movie or TV show and know
what he's watching?   **Yes / No**

Can he engage in a conversation? Does he talk
or mostly listen?   **Yes / No**

Does he still answer the telephone and
understand the interaction?   **Yes / No**

Does he talk on the telephone to friends?   **Yes / No**

Does he have friends that come over to visit
or would come over if the housing set up
were more favorable?   **Yes / No**

Dining Room

Can he sit up and feed himself or does
he need help?   **Yes / No**

Does he still have the manual dexterity
to wield a knife and fork or does he have
arthritis or other problems that prevent
him from using his hands well?   **Yes / No**

Does he have trouble chewing any foods?   **Yes / No**

Does he need dental work to assist with this?   **Yes / No**

Does he need anyone to cut up his food into
small pieces or to prepare soups or other
more liquid-type nourishment?   **Yes / No**

Kitchen
Can he prepare meals for himself?   **Yes / No**

Are these just small meals, a re-heated
dinner from the night before or actually
cooking from scratch?   **Yes / No**

Can he still use the microwave, toaster oven,
kitchen grill, or stove?   **Yes / No**

Can he purchase groceries at the store, or
must someone else drive him, or go there
in his place?   **Yes / No**

Can he prepare any special foods or dietary
supplements that his doctor has ordered?   **Yes / No**

Can he wash the dishes, either at the sink or
in a dishwasher?   **Yes / No**

Laundry
Can he organize, wash, and dry the laundry,
keeping the clothes in good order?   **Yes / No**

Bedroom
Does he still walk (ambulatory) or
is he in a wheelchair?   **Yes / No**

Does he need help in and out of bed?   **Yes / No**

Does he need assistance due to incontinence
issues (more frequent changing of your parent's
bedding and clothing, an increased need for
bathing or washing up, etc.)?   **Yes / No**

Is he easily frightened and needs someone
by his bedside?   **Yes / No**

Does he have a tendency to wander around
and needs someone to always keep an eye
on his whereabouts?   **Yes / No**

Does he need someone by his bedside to assure
administration of medication or
other treatments?   **Yes / No**

Bathroom
Can your parent get into and out of the
bath tub or shower?   **Yes / No**

Does he still understand a hot water vs.
cold water tap?   **Yes / No**

Does he still understand when the water
in the tub is too high, or that the surface
of the tub or floor could be slippery?   **Yes / No**

Will someone need to help him bathe,
either by securing him in place in the tub,
or actually cleaning him?   **Yes / No**

Does he need to be lifted or carried there?   **Yes / No**

Does he need assistance using the toilet?   **Yes / No**

Outside
Does your parent need assistance to go
outside for some sunshine?   **Yes / No**

Does he need someone to assist with
pushing a wheelchair? If so, does he need
an electric model or simply assistance?   **Yes / No**

Can he walk on sidewalks, grass, or
gravel without easily falling?   **Yes / No**

Can he go for walks down the block and
back alone or is there a danger that
he might wander and go missing?   **Yes / No**

Can he still participate in any outdoor
activities (jogging, walking the dog around
the block) without getting lost or disoriented?   **Yes / No**

Comments:

TIP 17

Consider Ways to Pay for Your Parent's Care

How to Figure Out Paying for Your Parent's Care

The subject of money always makes people tense. So, reading this section may upset you. The key is to be realistic about what your parent's situation is and what you can expect from yourself and others. Few of us are blessed with unlimited time, energy, or money. We have to make choices for the best solution we can find at the time. Do not feel guilty if your solution is not someone else's ideal. You are doing the best you can for your parent. Just do that, and everything else will be fine.

One of the potentially most useful websites I accessed, the Genworth Cost of Care Survey, was one linked on the United States' Health and Human Services office's **LongTermCare.gov** (https://longtermcare.acl.gov) website (that I had, in turn, located through a link on Medicare.gov). The Genworth site has a **Compare Long Term Care Costs Across the United States** webpage (https://www.genworth.com/about-us/industry-expertise/cost-of-care.html) that lists Daily, Monthly, and Annual costs for various kinds of long-term care, including: Homemaker Services Assistants, Home Health Aides, Home Caretakers, Adult Day Care, Assisted Living Facilities, Nursing Home Facilities (with Semi-Private and Private Room rates). Read this site. Get an idea of what the costs are. Then with the suggestions listed here, as well as your own ideas, start planning how you will pay for care for your parent.

Perhaps your circumstances dictate that there is really no choice, you have to use a particular caretaker or organization. Okay. I get that. I still maintain that by being aware of what's out there and what it will both give to your parent and take away from him, then maybe you can make the best choice possible within that framework.

Though some of my stories may make it sound as though my family had a lot of re-sources, in reality our options were as confined as many of yours, and in some ways, we are still recovering financially from some of our choices.

When you are confused or stumped and simply don't know what to do, start call-ing for help. Start with Medicare/Medicaid and/or the Social Security Administration. Remember, when it comes to the various government offices, your parent has sup-ported these services not only through his Medicare and Social Security deductions, but also through his taxes. Now that he is in need, he deserves to use their assistance. They have many well-informed people who are there to help. Let them help you.

Consider Ways to Save Money Through a Variety of Caretaker Setups

Family Members Fill-in as Caretakers

When your parent requires either no hands-on care or very little, it might be possible to setup a caretaking system that includes family members. The more care your parent requires, the more difficult it may be for a family member to be the one assisting your parent in his home. While they can, however, family members can contribute to your parent's care and save the family money. As I stated, filling in with family members works best at the lower levels. If your parent functions well and only requires someone to come by to remove snow, cut grass, etc., that's one thing. If your parent functions in the mid-level and needs meals cooked, but can still be at the house by himself, still that's a possible slot that a willing and appropriate family member could fill, at least for a while, if they have a schedule that will accommodate that situation. Beyond this level, however, it is best to have professionals, whether your parent continues to live at home or lives in a facility.

Hire a Day-Time Caretaker

Perhaps your family can be there for most things, but they can't be there to fix a healthy meal for morning and mid-day, or to remind mom or dad that it's time to handle things they can still do on their own like take their medication, or keep mom or dad from going out for a walk alone. Consider a Home Caretaker, Home Health Aide, or Homemaker Services Assistant. They can do some or all of these things, and the family members can take over when they return in the evening.

Hire a Live-in, Independent Caretaker for an "All-Included Price," Privately or Through a Service

If more care is required, consider keeping costs down and providing good care for your parent by hiring a live-in caretaker for your parent. I describe these caretakers as "independent," because they are not working for a nursing or other agency, they are working for themselves. One of the best, though hardest, things that we ever did was secure a live-in caretaker for my mom. We managed to find someone who would live in my mom's house, fix her meals—including soft and liquid meals made from fresh vegetables and other nutritious ingredients prepared daily, bathe her, dress her, do her hair, and care for her in the dignified and loving fashion she deserved. Because we provided the caretaker with a room, board (all of the caretaker's food), cable, and also made a car available since my mom was no longer driving her vehicle, we were able to negotiate a salary that we could manage. By paying the caretaker a salary rather than an hourly wage, we didn't have to worry about the cost of my mom's care going up if she stayed up one-hour too late and the caretaker had to look after her for that hour. The caretaker was there, in my mom's house, and on-duty around the clock. Therefore, she was there whenever she was needed. When my mom didn't need her care, the caretaker could watch TV, talk on the phone, or simply read a magazine in peace and quiet.

To arrange this caretaker situation, we used an online referral service to gather a list of potential candidates. That service listed candidate names, locations, credentials, and their philosophy—why they enjoyed being caretakers and how they approached their work. We then talked to several people on the phone. We performed in-person interviews. At first, we had to get over the fact that we didn't see a lot of people we wanted to leave alone with our mother. We persevered, however, and located someone we thought had the caretaking background and skill level we needed and the maturity we desired. We found our match. We financed this caretaker setup (as well as my mom's mortgage payment, the general upkeep of her home, the payment of her bills, etc.) with a combination of the money she had so diligently saved, our own funds, and in small ways that we somehow managed to work out as we needed them.

Therefore, if cost is a concern and you still want to provide one-on-one care for your parent, consider this arrangement. It might be a way to save money. Just be ready to screen, screen, screen and to do credential, reference, and background checks. Try to prepare by your parent's saving as much money ahead of time—in his retirement fund, for example—as possible.

Save Money but Protect Your Parent; Use Caution When People Are There in Your Absence

Be very careful with this kind of arrangement. You are deciding to put your parent, who may not be able to defend himself any better than a five-year old, in the exclusive care of another person. If you would not leave a young, defenseless child in this person's care, do not leave your parent in his or her care. Also, use these ideas to keep your parent safe:

- **Visit your parent's home frequently and unannounced**, so that if this person is partying during the day instead of caring for your parent, you know and you know fast.

- **Make hard, clear, and never to be violated rules about who the caretaker can have in the house**, you want the caretaker to be happy, but your parent's house is not a place for people to hang out. The caretaker's social life should happen on the weekends or on whatever days off he or she has and it should take place away from your parent's house. You will need to work out this part of the arrangement. Also, don't forget that you will need to arrange for care when the caretaker is away. (Let's put it this way, remember Mr. French, who was the manservant to the character Uncle Bill and then became caretaker for the three orphaned children in the old sitcom, *Family Affair*? Well, Mr. French did not party at Uncle Bill's apartment while Sissy, Buffy, and Jody were there. He socialized on his days off. It was the same with the character Alice on *The Brady Bunch*. Think of it that way.)

- **Make sure the caretaker never allows someone unauthorized to gain entry into your parent's house while you are gone** by saying things like: "I'm a relative . . ." or "She always lets me borrow . . ." If you haven't authorized someone to be there, they shouldn't be there. Period.

- **Make sure you have cameras in the home (ones not easily manipulated by others).** People have been assaulted and people have been mistreated in home care situations. Don't be naïve. Be smart if you choose this arrangement.

Medicare and Medicaid Benefits

At this writing, Medicare and Medicaid may not kick in for 24/7 care unless you are in a facility. You *may* only be eligible to receive visits for a limited number of hours; however, some care might be available. Even if the same person (the person from Medicare/Medicaid) cannot be there all day, every day, the assistance they give can save you some of the money you have to spend out of pocket. You need to check to see what services are available depending on the housing/living option you want. In addition, find out whether there is insurance you or your parent can carry as "gap" insurance to cover what your parent's current policy does not cover. Also, for more information and ideas, try the *Nursing Home Compare* information and the *Hospice Benefits* booklet available at Medicare.gov or call 1-800-MEDICARE (1-800-633-4227) or your State Medical Assistance (Medicaid) Office to get the most current information. I have not used these resources, but you may want to review them. Medicare/Medicaid offers various materials to explain their policies and help you.

https://www.medicare.gov/pubs/pdf/10153.pdf
http://www.medicare.gov/coverage/long-term-care.htm
https://www.medicare.gov/coverage/home-health-services.html

Additional Medical Insurance

Whether for you this is Medicare Gap insurance or an additional policy that your parent has just because, this insurance might pick up costs where your parent's Medicare ends. If your parent has a regular health insurance policy in addition to Medicare, then look on the back of the insurance card to find the member services number where you can call for advice. Perhaps if you simply tell them the problem, they will have a good solution, or at least tell you how to get started.

Life Insurance from a Departed Spouse

If one of your parents has already passed away, did that parent leave an insurance policy that could be used to supplement the cost of your surviving parent's care or living expenses? You need to check for any information you have from any of the insurance companies with which the departed parent dealt. (Also check with the Department of Veteran's Affairs if the departed parent was a vet and/or with the Social Security office—and you can do this whether or not the departed parent was a federal employee.)

If you go to check and you cannot find the name of an insurance company, or a policy number, or even exactly when or where any insurance policy might have been taken out, try the American Council on Life Insurers (ACLI), which is a Washington, D.C.-based lobbying and trade group. In November 2016, this group put out a press release announcing a new database from the National Association of Insurance Commissioners' (NAIC), called the **Lost Policy Locator Service**. See below for how to access this online service. It may be able to help you locate an existing policy, and the money it represents, whether or not you have the policy information.

- **American Council on Life Insurers (ACLI)** https://www.acli.com/Posting/NR16-041

- **National Association of Insurance Commissioners (NAIC)**
  Lost Policy Locator Service
  https://eapps.naic.org/life-policy-locator/#/welcome

Social Security Benefits

Get Your Social Security Administration Benefit Information

Ask your parent, if possible, or contact the Social Security Administration (SSA) about any benefits your parent has coming to him. If one of your parents has already passed away, there may be benefits due to the surviving spouse. Check into it. If your parent receives social security benefits already and has Medicare, then he can create a Social

Security account to get a benefit verification letter, as well as check his information, benefits, and earnings record.

- **Social Security Administration – Find Your Parent's Benefits**
  https://www.ssa.gov/onlineservices/.

- **Social Security Administration – Find a Local Office**
  Go to your computer, go online to this location: https://secure.ssa.gov/ICON/ main.jsp and then enter your zip code to find the nearest Social Security Administration office.

Get Assistance in Your Language

The Social Security Administration can even provide language interpreter services if you need them, so don't be afraid to contact them, even if language feels like a barrier. Call 1-800-772-1213. Currently for Spanish you press 7 and wait for a Spanish-speaking representative to come on the line. If you need a language other than English or Spanish, stay on the phone, do not push any buttons and wait for the operator to come on the line. When he does, have someone ask for the language you need.

Veteran Benefits

Obtain Your Veteran's Affairs Benefit Information

If your parent was a veteran, contact the Department of Veteran's Affairs (VA). The VA pays for certain service-related long-term care, and can provide at home nursing care and other services if your parent meets the requirements for these benefits. In addition, make sure you ask about the Housebound Aid and Attendance Allowance Program and the Veteran Directed Home and Community Based Services program (VD-HCBS).

Call 1-800-827-1000 or review the LongTermCare.gov website for more information: (https://longtermcare.acl.gov/medicare-medicaid-more/veterans-affairs-benefits.html).

Retirement and Pension Accounts

There are three different situations you need to check: 1.) your parent's retirement or pension accounts, 2.) a deceased parent's retirement or pension accounts, 3.) any special accounts set up to take the place of more traditional retirement or pension plans.

First, does your parent have a 401K (for profit employer) or 403B (nonprofit employer) retirement account fund or a pension that could assist with his care? Ask him or contact his former employers. Please note that sometimes people leave funds with past employers as well, not just with the last employer or the one from which he retired.

Second, if one of your parents has already passed away, did the deceased parent have a retirement or pension account that should be sending benefits to your living parent? Check with the deceased parent's former employer(s).

Third, if one of your parents was a homemaker, or perhaps self-employed, was there ever an account established so that she (or he) would at some time be able to draw retirement funds? Check into it.

Tax Benefits

Your Parent's Taxes

Consult an accountant on your parent's behalf—try H&R Block, Jackson-Hewitt, or one of the many other advertised tax preparation or assistance services. (I make no recommendations here; I'm just giving you a place to start. Ask your friends or your lawyer for recommendations.) and look into any tax benefits your parent may receive due to his age, physical condition, the status of his Alzheimer's or other dementia, or other factors.

Your Taxes

In addition, consult an accountant for yourself. You may be able to receive benefits if you pay for a portion of your parent's care. Perhaps your parent's dementia qualifies him to be designated as your dependent in some way. Ask. If available, these tax benefits could add just that amount that you cannot come up with in other ways.

Many factors go into calculating whether you, or your parent, will receive any tax benefits, and whether those benefits can assist your parent's housing/living situation. Start finding out.

Other Benefits

Just as there are school scholarships for kids who worked as golf caddies, or children of people who fought in a particular war, there are benefits that might be able to assist you and your parent in your fight against Alzheimer's or other dementia. Perhaps there are foundations that give some sort of supplemental assistance to people with your parent's medical issues. Perhaps doctors and scientists studying your parent's medical issues can offer assistance toward some part of your parent's care if he is participating in their study. Perhaps clubs or other organizations to which your parent belongs, such as churches or fraternal organizations, can assist. Some clubs have retirement homes for their members. Some clubs can put you in touch with other organizations that might be able to help. I don't know and you don't know either. This may take some research and you may not find anything at all. Still let your imagination and your research skills (or those of a good librarian) at least consider other possibilities.

TIP 18

Remember, It's Not Just Care; It's a Housing/Living Situation for Your Parent

How to Decide on Your Parent's Care

Before You Make Decisions about where Your Parent Will Be Cared for and Will Live, Think About These Things:

- **It's where your parent will spend every day, possibly for the remainder of his life.** Now, when it comes to your parent's care, he will no longer simply be going to a doctor's office and returning to his home, as all of us have done at one time or another since we were young children. No, your parent will eventually remain at this "doctor's office." Either his home will also become an examining room and perhaps at some point a hospital room, or he will move to another location where he will experience that same metamorphosis in his situation.

- **It's where you and the other family members will interact with your parent and live at least part of your own lives.** Your parent's care will take on a closeness and intimacy, both for him and for the entire family, that is unusual. You may have to have people outside the family around the house all of the time or you may go to visit your parent and have to get used to his roommate being there and sharing in your conversations.

Meals, which used to be just-grab-what-you-want-out-of-the-refrigerator-affairs, may become situations where a skilled nutritionist has to prepare special foods, or food must be eaten in a cafeteria-type atmosphere. None of these things are bad., but some or all of them will effect your family dynamic.

- **It's where both quiet people and more gregarious people will have to find their niche.** I have asked you to consider your parent's condition, as well as his ability to pay, now I am asking you to take into consideration the kind of person your parent is and keep that person in mind as you select what is best for your parent's overall health and well-being. Consider his likes and dislikes. Consider your likes and dislikes. For some people, being around other people is like a breath of fresh air and it makes them live a longer, happier existence. For other people, being able to have privacy and peace and quiet is equally as life affirming. Therefore, I am including a plea that you also, if at all possible and not detrimental to securing your parent's overall care, keep who your parent really is in mind as you consider the options.

- **It's a decision you, and possibly you alone, will have to live with, both now while your parent is living and later after he passes away.** One last thing, when it comes to your parent's care, remembering to listen to yourself becomes even more important. You are going to get criticism. Some people will wonder why on earth you are taking care of your parent at home. Other people will wonder why on earth you would ever consider putting your parent in a nursing home, when you're home all day with nothing to do. Here's something to consider: If they're not holding your parent's hand, cooking his food, or cleaning his house, then ignore them, because they do not know what it is to take care of your parent—not someone else's aunt's cousin's parent—your parent. And even if they are doing all of those things, you have been put in charge for a reason. It might have been that your parent designated you as his power of attorney or his guardian. It might have happened because of something else. Regardless, it's time now for you, along with those few others who will be caring for your parent in one way or another, to decide. Make sure it's a decision you can live with, not one someone else needs.

Select Your Parent's Best Housing/Living Option and an Appropriate Level of Care

How to Proceed

Understand the housing/living options available, understand the levels of care required, and then combine the two of these to come up with a caretaking setup for your parent.

Understand the Housing/Living Options

This section shows how to select a care option based on your parent's current health condition. How much care your parent needs is key. Remember the level of care your parent needs is often available in more than one living situation. For example, your parent may require adult day care; well, he can get that care either in his own home, at an Adult Day Care Center, or at a Respite Care facility. Keep this in mind.

Housing/Living Options

- **Option 1**: Your Parent Stays in His Own Home

- **Option 2**: Your Parent Moves in with You

- **Option 3**: Your Parent Moves in with Someone Else (preferably, one of your siblings)

- **Option 4**: Your Parent Moves into a Facility (i.e., Senior Living, Assisted Living, Nursing Home, or Hospice)

Understand the Levels of Care

Care means many things. Care includes everything from the need for a temporary stay in a rehabilitation facility to heal a broken leg, to needing someone to prepare meals in your home and drive you around while you go about your usual tasks, to needing assisted living facilities with medical services, to needing advanced medical care in a hospice.

Levels of Care

- **Temporary (Rehabilitation, Adult Day Care, Respite Care)**

- **Minimal (Senior Living)**

- **Moderate (Assisted Living, Nursing Home)**

- **Advanced (Nursing Home, Hospice)**

Use the Quick Guide to Putting Housing/Living Options and Levels of Care Together

Requires Temporary Care

Option 4 Rehabilitation Care
Option 4 Adult Day Care
Option 4 Respite Care

- **Right now, your parent needs a temporary option to deal with a specific heath issue rather than a permanent housing/living situation.** For example, if your parent has broken a leg or hip, and considerable convalescent care is required, you could seek a temporary stay in a rehabilitation (rehab) facility, rather than uprooting your parent permanently. During the time your parent is being treated for his temporary condition, you can make use of your parent's time away from his home to think about what you *will do* when a permanent housing/living situation change—such as either adding a caretaker to his current home or finding an appropriate assisted living, nursing home, or other facility in which he can live—is needed). (**Rehabilitation "Rehab" Care**)

- **You work from nine to five and need to keep your job, but you also want to make sure your parent is safe and well-cared for during the day.** Right now, your parent doesn't need a lot of hands-on care, but needs someone there with him. (**Adult Day Care**)

- **You could use a break from taking care of your parent to have some time to take care of yourself.** Maybe you have tickets to a once in a lifetime concert and want to go and enjoy yourself without worrying about your parent the entire time. (**Respite Care**)

Requires Minimal (If Any) Long-Term Care

Option 1 Stay at Home
Option 4 Senior Living Center

- **Your parent functions well and is happy where he is.** He can walk around without getting lost or confused; make small snacks and meals; converse with neighbors, friends, and strangers; drive a car, pay bills, operate the oven. He likes his neighbors and is glad to still have friends in the area. He requires assistance with lawn cutting, snow removal, help with carrying groceries, help driving on long road trips, but functions fine at daily tasks including moderate local driving. (**Stay at Home**)

- **Your parent functions just fine, but he never wants to mow a lawn or paint a fence again.** He'd like to live the good life for a change. He hopes to be able to fish and swim, maybe even get in a nature walk or two with some other like-minded seniors. (**Senior Living Center**)

Requires Moderate to Advanced Long-Term Care

Option 1+ Stay at Home with Assistance (i.e., Caretaking, Meal Program, such Meals-on-Wheels™, etc.)
Option 4   Assisted Living

Option 4   **Nursing Home**
Option 4   **Hospice**

- **If your parent still walks on his own, still reasons well and handles many tasks,** but his hand may tremble more than is good to be cooking at the stove, or his tendency to forget that food is on the stove or the door is wide open may require that someone else be there with him. Assistance can include, but is not limited to: preparing meals, ensuring he takes his medication, accompanying him on walks. **(Stay at Home with a Caretaker and Meal Program)** or **(Assisted Living)**

- **If your parent can no longer move as fast, fix his meals, or have the lively conversations he used to have,** but he's still aware of most things around him. If your parent uses a wheelchair, for example, perhaps he wielded his chair just fine on his own before, but now he's more tired when he does it or he finds he needs to be or prefers to be pushed. Your parent may move around the house slowly on his own or he may even be confined to bed. Your parent will likely require assistance with most, if not all, day-to-day needs such as bathing, toileting, and feeding himself. He may have good days when he can do more things; he may have bad days when he needs more help. He cannot be left alone. This level of care could be accommodated at a residential facility. This level of care could also, however, be accommodated at home if an appropriate care provider is available. Appropriate "stay at home" care here could be a live-in caretaker situation or a two-caretaker situation, with each caretaker handling a twelve-hour shift and neither of them living at home with your parent. **(Stay at Home with a Caretaker—possibly a live-in caretaker—and a Meal Program)** or **(Nursing Home)**

- **If your parent requires assistance at his bedside,** turning so that bedsores are avoided, assistance with all tasks indicated in the last bullet, a level of care that amounts to twenty-four-hours a day, seven-days a week (24/7), plus the administration of medication for pain control, and/or feeding by feeding tube, if necessary. Sometimes this level of care can be accommodated at home. Most times, this level of care must be handled at a residential facility. (**Stay at Home with At-Home-Hospice care from a hospice provider, and possibly a Meal Program**), or (**Stay at Home with a live-in caretaker skilled in serious nursing care, and possibly a Meal Program**), or (**Hospice**)

Use the Detailed Guide to Putting Housing/Living Options and Levels of Care Together

This section will give you more details about the care options. For example, not only will it connect the level of care your parent needs to a housing/living situation, but it will also suggest the people for whom each option is a "best choice," what you need to think about regarding the dementia, and what you need to think about regarding your own or a family member's participation.

Sometimes, you start with an aging parent who really does not need medical help, but rather needs help around the home. Other times, you start with a parent who is already displaying more advanced symptoms, requiring more care and perhaps a change in living circumstances. That's why I have included detailed descriptions of all four housing/living situations introduced previously:

Option 1: Your Parent Stays in His Own Home

Description

This is my preference, and it is what I did for my mom. And it can be an especially attractive option if your parent's home is already paid for. It's not easy, and though I would choose it again, I do not recommend it for everyone. I did it because all my life my mom asked us all to make sure she remained at home and not at a facility. She felt this way for many reasons. She was older and grew up with the idea of living out the rest of her life at home, surrounded by her family. She wanted to be able to look at the trees she had grown up with and glance out her window at relatives who lived nearby. She was also a registered nurse and knew what was and was not available and possible at most senior facilities. She knew some were excellent and some were not. And she knew most were regimented. She did not want a regimented life. She wanted to live

117

the way she always had: independently. She did not want to eat at times designated by others. She did not want to have to participate in activities or join groups that just were not for her—required gym class in school had been enough for her. She wanted to live her older life the way she had lived her younger life: as an autonomous person. I, in turn, wanted to make sure that is what she got to do. (My dad was being cared for at home when he died of cancer. My mom wanted to be cared for at home as well.)

An additional step you might want to take while considering having your parent stay in his own home is to familiarize yourself with current technologies that will make this option more feasible. For example, start with the HGTV.com article, recommended in the tip on Use Technology to Protect Your Parent's Well-being, titled *Aging In Place Home Technologies*[19]. Also refer to the tip "Help Your Parent Maintain His Home for ideas on how to improve your parent's (and any caretaker's) stay in the home.

Consider If

- Is the old neighborhood—the one you grew up in and the one in which your parent still lives—a good one, with low crime and well-liked neighbors? Then perhaps option number one—your parent's own home, with some adjustments—might be the best fit.

- Were your parent's activities mainly solo events or those involving mostly family and very close friends? If so, option one might be best.

- Does your family have a tradition of caring for its elderly or infirmed members at home? Are you prepared (or willing to get prepared) to do what is necessary to provide good at home care for now and/or as your parent's illness progresses in the future? If so, consider Option 1.

If Your Parent Is Still Functioning Well

Having your parent stay in his own home doesn't have to mean living alone. It can mean living with a new roommate. It also might mean having a relative move in with

---

19 "Aging In Place Home Technologies," HGTV.com, accessed March 22, 2017, http://www.hgtv.com/remodel/mechanical-systems/aging-in-place-home-technologies.

him. You could get a sibling or a grandchild to live with him. Perhaps someone who's going to school and needs inexpensive housing, or perhaps a relative making a career transition who could use reduced rent and life with someone who still recalls how to bake cookies from scratch. They could help each other. Just make sure that the terms of the living situation are clear from day one.

If Your Parent Requires More Serious Care

Having your parent stay in his own home could even mean getting a live-in caretaker to be there full-time with your parent, which is what I did. This last suggestion might seem beyond your means, but then again it might not be. There are many good, professional caretakers who either need or are willing to accept a live-in situation and would be willing to work with you to come to an agreement that will suit and benefit you both. Also, the two-caretaker situation that I mentioned earlier, with each caretaker handling a twelve-hour shift and neither of them living at home with your parent, might be something else to consider. Over the course of my mother's illness, I used various forms of care: an at home nursing service called A-1 Action Nursing, a caretaker service called Care.com, and personal arrangements with family members and nursing professionals that I knew (and I am grateful to all of these people because they made my life easier and my mom's life safer and richer).

Dementia Challenges—How Does this Option Help or Hurt?

Another reason I support option one, staying in his own home, is that dementia patients retain a great deal of information from long-term memory and often less from short-term memory. Your parent may remember his neighborhood sidewalks the ones he strolled along with his wife when you kids were young, but he will likely forget those in your or your sibling's new neighborhood, or those surrounding a facility. This fact can put your parent in jeopardy if he is out alone or is starting to wander and getting to places with no idea where he is or how to get back home. Therefore, keeping your parent in a stable location (his current home) with a sibling or other close relative moving in; a live-in, paid caretaker; or two caretakers handling shifts, might be preferable. (Though please remember that any good facility will have a system in place to monitor and watch your parent.)

Your Challenges—How Does this Option Help or Hurt?

Do you need to visit every day because your parent's health is very bad, or will a visit once a week or so suffice? If you did need to visit every day, could you? How much will that add to your gasoline bill, wear and tear on your car, or the necessity to bring work home each night to complete it because you'll need to leave the office a little sooner?

Another thing to consider with this care is what happens next. For instance, will you eventually decide to move your parent into a facility (because you would prefer a facility as opposed to having twenty-four-seven care or hospice care handled at home)? If so, that might make a difference to you when you think about whether you will begin your parent with care at home. In that case, perhaps moving to a facility sooner makes sense. If, however, you would definitely consider having whatever long-term care your parent needs given in the home, then orienting your parent to the people who will be around him might make sense for you. If you do begin with care at home, your parent may be able to become comfortable with and trust caretakers while he is still fully cognizant. This situation could make it easier for him. When his dementia becomes more advanced, he will already know and like the people around him caring for him daily. Your parent will already have gotten used to caretakers he learned to like and trust while he was better. Think of it from both of these angles and see what feels most beneficial to your parent and practical and safe to you. Please read the section on facilities (Option 4), and the tips that follow on twenty-four-seven care (which provides care twenty-four-hours a day, seven-days a week) and hospice care (which provides care for those with terminal illnesses or conditions). Lastly, when it comes to hospice care, remember to make sure that any organization you contact to provide such care guarantees that they (the hospice staff) will be there, in your home, and you and your family will not have to act as bedside nurses to your (then terminally ill) parent.

Option 2. Your Parent Moves in with You

Description

If your parent lives with you, it will be similar to his staying in his own home. Your parent is familiar with you; your home has probably been a place he has visited many times and in which he feels comfortable. And even if that's not true, and your parent has only been there once, your presence will make it feel like home.

In addition, if you ever decide to move from your current home to another home, take your parent with you. He is now part of *your* family. Please let him remain a part of it.

Consider If

- Do you get along with your parent? If not, do not put yourself in an option number two situation—moving your parent into your own home. It will hurt you and your parent.

- Do you have time to visit your parent at least once a week, if he or she does not live with you, but rather is in a facility? if no, reconsider option two, which would locate your parent conveniently, i.e., where you live.

Dementia Challenges—How Does this Option Help or Hurt?

One major caution when moving your parent in with you: orient him to your area and then make sure you are with him when he is outside. If his confusion now includes memory loss and/or a tendency to wander, *you must always remember to accompany your parent whenever he is outside.* Dementia patients retain a great deal of information from long-term memory and often less from short-term memory. The home you grew up in with him is in his long-term memory. Your new condo or 10-year old house in the suburbs may be in short-term memory, and thus, easily forgotten by him. Even if he doesn't wander, he may walk a couple of blocks and then realize he doesn't know the street names as well as he thought. He might then have no idea where he is, how to get back to your home, or even what your street address is so that others could help him. So, care must be taken when it comes to allowing your parent outside on his own. He needs to be accompanied, even if it's just your holding his arm as you both take a relaxing stroll around the block. Remember this.

Your Challenges—How Does this Option Help or Hurt?

Do you need to work at home too, and do you require peace and quiet to do that? Can you have that with your parent there? Will your parent's presence substantially alter your home life? Is yours the best home for your parent, or would another relative with a first-floor bedroom or no stairs be a better choice at this time?

Option 3. Your Parent Moves in with Someone Else

Description
If your parent lives far away from you, you need special strategies to keep him safe and to know—not just give yourself false reassurance—that he will be all right. If you have a sibling or close relative who lives near your parent, then consider that person as a possible live-in choice for mom or dad. This situation should be one that is almost the same as him living with you.

Consider If

- Is there a sibling who wants your parent with him? (Be honest about whether you think that sibling would take good care of your parent. This is not about loving your sibling; it's about his or her ability to become a caretaker to someone who genuinely needs care.) If you can say, "Yes, my sibling would be okay at this," or "Yes, I trust my sibling to hire a good reliable caretaker," then try option three.

Dementia Challenges—How Does this Option Help or Hurt?
Having people you know take care of you is better than having strangers with no social or familial connection to you. If you have a parent who is a bit gruff on his best days, then family might trump a caretaking service in getting him to be more cooperative. (Of course, most trained caretakers have dealt with worse and should be trained to handle your parent.)

Your Sibling or Close Relative's Challenges—How Does this Option Help or Hurt?
Is the person who will be living with your parent capable of caring for himself *and* your parent at this or future stages while your parent remains in that person's home? For

example, can he handle such things as obtaining a special bed or other items that your parent may need? Would you trust that person with a five-year-old child who didn't speak your language? (If not, forget it right now!) If this is a family member, will his caring for your parent end his relationship with the parent or with you, either because he is argumentative, impatient, selfish, undependable, or he just has a difficult history with your parent or the family? If this is not an immediate family member, what makes you comfortable giving him this level of responsibility? You need to know the person you're counting on and whether you have a reasonable expectation that he can take on these caretaking tasks.

Your Challenges—How Does this Option Help or Hurt?
If you live too far away to visit your parent frequently, you are not a bad son or daughter. You are one of millions who struggle every day in our highly mobile society. There are ways to stay in touch anyway. There are computer and cell phone applications— for example, FaceTime (FaceTime.com) or Skype (Skype.com)—that allow you to see the person you are talking to and for that person to see you. (And if you don't understand what FaceTime and Skype are, where to find them, or how to use them, visit the websites listed in this paragraph.)

In addition, you can take baby pictures of yourself when you go visit your parent and slowly explain that you are the child in the photo. There are lots of ways to connect to your parent frequently. Only your imagination will stop you on this one.

Option 4. Your Parent Regularly Goes to or Moves into a Facility

Description

Temporary Residential Facilities

- **Adult Day Care** refers to temporary care, usually hourly or daily (for example, nine to five when the family is at work), where the individual returns home each evening.

- **Rehabilitation (Rehab)** These facilities are a sub-group of the hospital or assisted living type facility. They offer temporary care in a residential facility for those presenting injuries or illnesses that can be difficult for family members to handle, such as a broken leg or hip. They are not places for your parent to stay long-term, nor do they offer hospice or end-of-life care. Instead, these facilities are meant to handle specific issues, temporarily. They can be used to supplement the other kinds of facilities discussed here.

- **Respite Care** refers to temporary care, sometimes similar to hourly or daily adult day care—where the individual returns home at night, other times similar to short-term stay care—where the individual remains at the respite facility for a specific number of days. The purpose of respite care is to provide short-term relief to the caretaking family, whose parent is receiving hospice-level (terminally ill) care, as well as for others seeking caretaking relief. This could mean free time for the family to perform the monthly grocery shopping, time for her to go to the hairdresser's alone, or time for him to visit his own doctor. The idea is to give the caretaker a break and allow him or her to return to the parent refreshed and ready to resume his or her caretaking duties. This type of care is also useful to cover full-time caretakers who must take vacation breaks and is useful as part of a family's complete caretaking set up.

Permanent Residential Facilities

One Caution

Care options are usually selected according to the level or stage at which the patient's condition presents itself, not what the condition may or may not become in the future; however, you must consider such issues when it comes to long-term health care planning, especially if that planning includes locking yourself into any housing/living arrangements with others or with facilities.

Senior Living, Assisted Living, Nursing Home, and Hospice Care

- **Senior living** refers to condos, apartments, or even single-family homes in "fifty-five and over" communities. These are usually planned communities that offer amenities such as easy access to grocery stores, dry cleaning, hair-dressers, and other daily conveniences. Often a shuttle bus is available to connect residents with these services. There is also usually a clubhouse-type facility that offers activities in which residents may participate, as well as or-ganized exercise classes and social events. Here, the resident is running his or her own life with no restrictions. **Be careful of and aware of the uses of the terms "Senior living" and "Assisted living."** Some senior-living facili-ties function more like assisted living or nursing home facilities, with more stepped-up care and monitoring. Make sure to check the details so that you get the kind of facility you want.

- *Assisted living* refers to complexes similar to those offered in senior living de-scribed above but with the added amenity of on-site medical monitoring or medical access. There are also usually personnel available to assist you if you need assistance in your day-to-day activities; however, you are usually free to move about and come and go as you need to. The resident is running his or her own life, with a few restrictions. Sometimes, assisted living facilities have a medical "step-up" type of option with which you can have more bedside and other medical assistance as your condition warrants, so that as your illness progresses, your assisted living facility becomes virtually a nursing home for you. (Ask whether there is an opportunity for shifting from assisted living to a nursing home level of care while remaining at the same facility, if it is needed.) These facilities usually have formal systems for monitoring your condition and whereabouts as wanted and as necessary. Consider trying a Place for Mom, www.aplaceformom.com, 1-866-333-1356 (which you may recognize from their spokesperson, Joan Lunden), which frequently advertises on TV as a service that can assist you in locating assisted living as well as nursing home facilities, as well as the CCRC, PACE, and HCBS programs described under Medicare/Medicaid— Additional Care Opportunities later in this tip.

- *Nursing homes* often have the amenities noted above, with the facility looking either like a large home, an apartment complex or community, or sometimes like a hospital. The residents at this type of facility require and are afforded additional medical services. Often, when assisted living facili-ties have a medical "step-up" type of choice where you can have more bed-side and other medical assistance as your condition warrants, that resulting facility either resembles or actually is a nursing home. Thus, there can be a relationship between the assisted living and nursing home facilities, and sometimes the same complex can house both choices. Therefore, a nursing home facility can resemble an apartment complex or a hospital floor, depending on the services the resident requires. Nursing home facilities will not only monitor your medical condition, but also will track your whereabouts. There will be limitations about when and under what conditions you can leave the premises. This restriction will be true for all residential medical facilities. (Try using the *Nursing Home Compare* information on Medicare. gov or reading the Medicare/Medicaid online booklet entitled, *Your Guide to Choosing a Nursing Home or Other Long-Term Care*, available at Medicare. gov. I have not used it, but it may be worth a review. Also, try ElderCare.org and AARP's Caregiver information, which I have sampled or a Place for Mom, www.aplaceformom.com, which frequently advertises on TV, as well as the CCRC, PACE, and HCBS programs described under Medicare/Medicaid— Additional Care Opportunities later in this tip.)

- *Hospice* **refers both to a facility (building) and a type of care**. A **hospice facility** is a building like a nursing home and it provides appropriate end-of-life care for terminally ill patients. **Hospice care**, is specifically geared to terminally ill patients, but it doesn't necessarily occur at a hospice facility. Hospice care *can* occur at a hospice facility, but it also can occur in the patient's home, at a nursing home, or at another similar type facility. This level of care is entered at some time when a serious illness has become terminal, usually the last six months of life. It usually involves constant monitoring, close access to nursing staff, and a focus on pain prevention and pain control. It provides care for all ongoing illnesses and symptoms. It is advanced care specifically to keep the patient as comfortable as possible during this stage of illness. (Refer to the *Hospice Benefits* booklet available at Medicare.gov. I have not used it, but you may want to check it out.)

Benefits of Facilities

Some people love the country-club or sleep-away-camp atmosphere of senior living and assisted living facilities. Many such facilities have residents dine together in a dining hall, offer plenty of activities from crafts to swimming, and provide a ready group of people to get to know. Residents can live close to all of this and just walk over, so there is no need to drive. Snow is shoveled, repairs are handled, and that leisurely lifestyle people talk about can be easily at hand. There are doctors available for those with medical issues. There are facilities that provide for those with specific health issues, such as Alzheimer's or other dementia.

Drawbacks of Facilities

Residential facilities are great places for the right person. If your parent was not a joiner before, perhaps this would give him the opportunity to do so in a supportive atmosphere and to take advantage of options to remain in his private rooms when socializing is not desired. Still, not everyone will be comfortable with this arrangement, so keep that in mind as you plan. Not everyone wants to socialize with his neighbors all day long and to have to see them at dinner each night. If your parent prefers the company of you and your children or a quiet walk with one of his neighbors, this might not be the best atmosphere for him. Staying in his own home and close to old neighbors, or with you, a sibling, or other close relative might be preferable. (Non-residential facilities—adult day care, for example—for as long as your parent's condition allows it, might be a more reasonable choice if your parent is uncomfortable with being away with others all of the time.)

Consider If

1. Be cautious about option four—moving into a facility—and *do not force your parent* into an option-four situation. Facilities are social places. Your parent may not have a private room. Your parent may be required to spend hours in an activity or lounge area with others he doesn't know. Consider these things. Quiet and private people do not suddenly become joiners when you put them in a facility. Quiet or private people need to be shown respect and consideration for who they are as these decisions are made. (Even Hospice-level care can be provided for in your parent's home. Please consider this option and if you do, make sure it is carried out with the most professional hospice [acute-care] caretakers they have.)

2. Is your parent a joiner—someone who needs to have people around, someone who had exercise walks, regular shopping outings, movie dates, golf

outings, bridge club, dinners, or vacations, where everyone was invited and welcomed? Then, option four might be a good one.

3. Do you have time to visit your parent at least once a week, if he or she does not live with you, but rather is in a facility? If you don't, can someone else look in on your parent? If yes, consider option four.

4. Is your parent very ill and in need of constant and professional care? Then do not be afraid to select one of the appropriate choices under option four. There are good facilities out there that will take good care of your parent. It might be the best thing for you *and* for him.

Dementia Challenges—How Does this Option Help or Hurt?

There is also the dementia issue to consider. Depending on the progress of your parent's dementia, he may not be able to take advantage of many of the benefits of a particular facility. Assisted living can give your parent the best of both worlds: a chance to have a facility that caters to his age group and provides support and activities within easy reach and a chance to be monitored and cared for with regard to his dementia issues. It also provides the sometimes much-needed relief to the family, who often struggle to continue their own lives in the midst of what often feels like a roller coaster of crises. (Mom had a good day yesterday. Mom is having a bad day today.)

You need to know where to place your parent. Your doctor and the checklist can help here. It's one thing to be in a senior living or assisted living situation when you can walk around, manage your own affairs, and the issue is a desire to enjoy retirement, not shovel snow anymore, or to easily enjoy the activities you love. It's quite another thing to be in this senior living or assisted living atmosphere when you may no longer be able to enjoy the craft class because you can no longer participate without assistance, or where you may not even understand what is going on, or where you are, or when someone is going to come for you.

Your Challenges—How Does this Option Help or Hurt?

Facilities Require that You Participate

Visit the Facility
Before your parent goes there, you go. Check out the facility thoroughly. Show up un-expectedly. Observe the place as a visitor before you even consider it for your parent. If you know people who have used it, ask them what their experience was and observe their expressions, not just their words. Look and see past the obvious impression the facility wants you to have. Are there patients in the halls? How are they dressed? Are they in pajamas at noon, or has someone washed them up and helped them get to an activity? How do the hallways and rooms look and smell? Clean and neat, though maybe a little lived in, or like they need a good scrubbing? How many patients look incoherent? How many, though they may have problems, look lively? If you are given appropriate access to current residents, are the patients themselves open or hesitant to talk to you? Do not try to convince yourself it's a good place without evidence—consistent, unquestionable evidence—to that fact. Or if you're a "gut feeling" kind of person, then make sure your gut feels calm and satisfied.

Plan to Visit Often
Do not place your parent in a facility with the idea that you no longer have to be involved. Your time requirement should lessen, but you need to continue to be avail-able to visit and check in on what's going on, how your parent is being treated, and how he is adjusting to life there. The minute the facility does not live up to some-thing, call them on it. If your parent looks consistently unhappy, talk to the appropri-ate staff at the facility. See what they suggest, and keep an eye out for whether there is improvement.

If your parent looks ill cared for, has sustained an injury, or is frightened, call the police if it is an emergency, and wait there until the police arrive. If it is not an emer-gency, call a lawyer, and let the lawyer protect your parent (by contacting appropriate authorities, finding another place for your parent to live, and removing him immediately from the current facility) and protect you (by handling issues regarding any money you have invested in the current facility). Trust your gut about what's bad enough. Look in the phone book (hardcopy or on the Internet), check out your local college's legal aid office, or watch your TV for an ad. Good legal help isn't always in a skyscraper in an expensive part of the city. There are law firms that specialize in cases involving nursing homes and other such facilities. They will likely take your case on a contingency basis, which means you will pay a portion of your money to them once they win your case. Look into it if there are problems, especially if mistreatment is at all an issue. Lawyer up and get your parent taken care of.

You cannot change a bad place into a good one. This is one of the main reasons that your parent needs your continued presence and participation in his care. Just keep your eyes open, and you'll be fine—and so will your parent.

If a facility is involved, you need to check it out thoroughly, continue to check it out, and go there frequently, whenever you can, or have someone whose opinion you trust go there in your place. Use the five-year-old test. Would you take a five-year-old to live away from home with strangers and only call once a week and see him only once a month? No? Then don't do that to a parent who has dementia. Your parent needs to see you frequently to remember your name and who you are to him. Your parent needs to feel loved frequently, because he may have forgotten that you visited him yesterday or last week. Your parent needs someone to listen to him—and someone to speak for, fight for, and look out for him. Your parent needs someone to make sure he is okay—that is, someone to see with his own eyes, not via some secondhand report from staff, that your parent's skin looks good, his eyes are clear, he is not sedated all day long to keep him quiet, and that he is not touched roughly or threatened or abused in any way—and that he is treated with dignity, respect, and care. Do not assume that nice people will not lose their tempers with your parent or resort to various less-than-optimal means to control him.

If You Can't Participate, (Though They Don't Require It) You Should Find Someone Else Who Can

As mentioned earlier, if you don't live close enough to visit your parent frequently, you are not a bad son or daughter, but you do need make sure that some other responsible person is there to visit and check on your parent's condition, as well as the staff treatment of your parent, and not only advocate for him, but also hold his hand and help keep his spirits up. So, make sure that you arrange for someone to do these things.

Also, of course, remember to use FaceTime® (FaceTime.com or Apple.com) or Skype® (Skype.com) to remain in contact with your parent. These are computer applications that allow you to see the person you are talking to—and allow him to see you. You can use these on a computer or a cell phone, as I have mentioned before. Maybe the friend that is helping you out by checking-in on your parent can also help him with one of these applications when he or she visits.

Additional Resources

These resources were suggested on the Memorial Sloan-Kettering website. I performed searches on each website to give them a try. See my results below:

1. **A Place for Mom**
   www.aplaceformom.com
   or
   http://www.joanlunden.com/a-place-for-mom
   1-855-707-5011 or 1-866-333-1356

   o   Do you remember Joan Lunden, from her TV news anchor days on *Good Morning America*? I would give a service she recommends a try. I searched A Place for Mom's website and found that they provide information on senior housing, including senior living, independent living, nursing homes, Alzheimer's Care, 55+ Apartments, and Respite Care. Their information includes costs, services, and amenities available.

2. **AARP Caregiving**
   www.aarp.org

   o   I found some very useful articles and other interesting resources worth checking out (https://search.aarp.org/gss/everywhere?q=AARP%20 Caregiving&intcmp=DSO-SRCH-EWHERE).

3. **Eldercare Locator**
www.eldercare.gov
1-800-677-1116

   ○ Eldercare.gov is a website from the U.S. Administration on Aging, under the Department of Health and Human Services (https://aoa.acl.gov/). For Eldercare.gov, I performed a sample search for resources. I searched for resources in the 02134-zip code (the Boston area--just a zip code I remembered from the old *Zoom* PBS show) and 92121 (the San Diego area—an area I've contacted before). The result? I received four categories of resources for each search: 1.) Information and Assistance, 2.) Area Agencies on Aging, 3.) Aging and Disability Resource Centers, and 4.) State Agency on Aging, with at least one resource listed in each category. The contact information for each resource included the street address, website, contact e-mail, office phone, information phone, TTY phone, languages they speak, a description of the services they give, special notes on additional services that might be of interest, their hours of operation, and a map with directions. To me, this says that this is a resource worth trying.

4. **Healthinaging.org**
www.healthinaging.org

   ○ For Heathinaging.org, which is a website created by the American Geriatrics Society's Health in Aging Foundation, I reviewed the website and found not only a great deal of information for caregivers—they have a quiz to assess caregiver stress, as well as articles on caregiver health, and caregiver burnout—but also a source of how-to instructions for finding a good nursing home. This is another site you really should visit, and often.

5. **Medicare/Medicaid—Additional Care Opportunities**
LongTermCare.gov
www.medicare.gov
www.medicaid.gov

- ○ Within the Assisted Living and Nursing Home website areas, three long-term care opportunities offered through Medicare/Medicaid stood out. For any of these programs, read more online at medicare.gov, contact Medicaid at your State Medical Assistance Office, or access Medicare's long-term care services page at LongTermCare.gov.

- **Programs for All-Inclusive Care for the Elderly (PACE)**—PACE is not about your parent's going to a nursing home or other facility. Its goal is to get your parent the care he needs where he is now, in his own community. This care may or may not require that your parent uses a PACE-preferred doctor. Read more online.

- **Home and Community-based Service 1915 (c) (HCBS) Waivers**—HCBS Waivers are offered by most states and they are for receiving long-term care in your home or community, rather than in a facility. Read more online.

- **Continuing Care Retirement Communities (CCRC)**—CCRCs offer a variety of care/housing living situations, from what they call "independent living units" to assisted living facilities, to nursing homes, all located in the same community. Contact 1-202-587-5001 to find out more.

TIP 19

Understand Twenty-four-Seven Care (24/7)

How to Think about Twenty-four-Seven (24/7) Care

What Is Twenty-four-Seven Care?

Twenty-four-Seven Care is short for "Twenty-four-hours a day, seven-days a week care (24/7)" and it can mean a lot of things. It can mean that the person has a tendency to leave his eyeglasses in the refrigerator and needs someone there to fetch them, make his meals, answer the door and the phone, and get his favorite shows on the TV. It can also mean that he is confined to bed and requires turning, assistance with toileting, feeding, and so forth. The level of care required will help narrow your choice of services. In either case, there are residential options that can accommodate you, whether you prefer the idea of your parent staying in his own home, yours, someone else's, or residing in a facility of some kind, such as an assisted living facility or a nursing home.

Twenty-four-Seven Care – at Home or in a Facility

Despite my tendency to stress the stay-in-his-own-home-and-have-others-live-with-him-if-necessary option, I would suggest, for more severe illnesses or the final stages, that you strongly consider having your parent in a facility or having an at-home hospice provider that, when the time comes, can *guarantee* its presence at the home bedside for all necessary care. You need someone who will be willing and able to give all end-stage pain medications. You need someone who knows how to move a patient properly with the least amount of discomfort for the patient. You need someone who can handle a feeding tube if there is one. You need someone who is trained at calmly focusing on your parent. And most importantly, you need people who can be fresh each shift and awake and available at 2:00 a.m. and at your parent's side. A family member, who is probably not a medical professional, cannot help but focus on being upset that he must administer a shot. He cannot help but be concerned that he will not remember the instructions shown him or that he will hurt the parent because he doesn't really know what he's doing after being shown how to administer a needle one time.

Be prepared with a choice of care and a specific facility to give that care, because the announcement that you need to give your parent 24/7 care is going to be a surprise. Know what you will have to pay, what any insurance or Medicare that your parent has will cover, and whether you must liquidate your parent's assets for him to be accommodated in either a public or a private facility. I do not know; you need to find out for yourself. Getting your parent into the facility that you want him to be in often takes knowledge and lead time. Navigating these issues may require that you talk to your local area's social services office, Medicare or Medicaid, your parent's doctor, and an appropriate representative at the facility in which you are interested.

The Suddenness of 24/7 Care

My mom's then current caretaker and I took my mom to a local hospital emergency room when she began not eating and showing some other signs of illness. After two weeks in the hospital, we were given one day's notice of when she would be discharged and told at that time she would need 24/7 care. We were told not to worry, that a social worker would contact us with assistance. This assistance consisted only of a list of nursing home facilities in the immediate area of the hospital. That's it. The social worker was not available to make calls on our behalf, talk to us about our options, or discuss how to go about setting up care, or any of the things that I expected. (Granted, I have never worked with a social worker before, so perhaps that is the normal situation and she was doing all she could do for us.) The hospital social worker could only offer us a list of nursing homes, which were available primarily to residents of the county where the hospital was located. Though less than half an hour's drive from us, it was not the county in which my mom resided. Thus, we couldn't use any of the nursing homes on the list. In addition, the current caretaker was not available to provide the level of care that my mother would now require. So immediately, I was without any care for my mom and with a requirement for 24/7 care hanging over my head. This is a long way of saying that you need to make sure you understand what residential, financial, or other qualifications you must meet in order to access the services your parent will need. Furthermore, you need to have a plan in place for them before you need it.

We could not find a nursing home we liked to even take my mom and get her through that first month of needing intense care to survive. When my mom was discharged from the hospital that next day, after much scrambling, we did locate a firm that made two full-time nursing assistants available, with each prepared to take a twelve-hour shift with my mom. With this level of care, she required over $10,000 in out-of-pocket expenses for nursing care that first month. We had no idea whether social services, Medicare/Medicaid, or other offices might have been able to help us with at least some of this expense. Though I did eventually learn that Medicare could have covered some of the expense, but only with temporary, occasional care for a few hours a week.

Things You Don't Expect with 24/7 Care

We had to learn to have other people in the house and attending to my mom around the clock. These things may seem trite, but if you're not as organized as you should be, here are some of the other things we had to get used to. The nurses needed to keep my mom's room, especially clean, so they needed items they could use to accomplish that. They needed a place next to my mother to sit and rest, because they couldn't stand for a twelve-hour shift. They needed one spot, not several, stocked with clean linens and a place for the oxygen tank to stand. Just be aware and be considerate. Also, remember that they are in your home all day, possibly without access to a car, (since they may have arrived via bus, or subway, or a ride). They are, for lack of better words, stuck in your house all day. Remember that they need reasonable breaks. Remember that they are not working next to a 7-Eleven® store or a McDonald's® restaurant and offer them some food and something to drink. No, they are not your guests, but my mother worked as a private-duty nurse on occasion and such niceties were always appreciated by her.

We had excellent nursing assistance and after one full month we were able to step down from two full-time nursing assistants to one nursing assistant, doing only a twelve-hour shift. The family filled in for the other twelve hours. This was when our caretaking journey really began. It was three years after I took my mom's keys. It was one of the worst periods of my life.

Do not let this happen to you. Have a place already picked out. Have a plan for how this intense care, if necessary, will fit into your overall life and finances. If the care becomes permanent rather than transitional, be prepared for that too.

TIP 20

Understand Hospice Care

How to Think about Hospice Care

When Hospice Care Starts

Hospice care is usually not available until the person is within the last six months of life, depending on the situation. This is a medical determination. Either your parent's doctor or the hospice doctor will make that determination based on an examination of the patient. This status kicks in to provide the most serious (acute) care for your parent. It is not to be feared. It is a means for your parent to have the right medication to control pain and a level of care to support where he is in medical transition. This is also usually when financial assistance from Medicare/Medicaid becomes available, but please confirm that this is the case for the time, exact diagnosis, and situation that you face. Go to the Medicare.gov website and search for the *Hospice Benefits* booklet in their Medical Publications area.

Different Kinds of Hospice Care

All hospice care is not the same. Some organizations provide not only hands-on medical care, but also music therapy, body massage, and other services that give the patient a sense of peace and comfort. Ask about these as well.

Details You MUST Know

If your parent is currently staying in a home situation and you will have him receiving hospice care there:

1. Will your parent be moved to a facility as his condition worsens?
2. If so, where and when can you go see it?
3. If not and all care will be given at home, will round-the-clock personnel be available, or will you have to call if you need someone?
4. If you have to call, what does that entail? Will someone come and be present at the home, immediately? If not immediately, then when? For how long? Under what circumstances?
5. Will the hospice give any and all end-stage medications for pain relief or feeding (feeding tubes), or will family members be responsible for administering these?

My Experience

Hospice care for us at home was sometimes difficult (and not quite what we expected). We couldn't have personnel there every moment that we wanted them there. We had to give medications, and though it was under strict orders and supervision, *we* were sometimes the on-site medical personnel for our parent, which is not what I had wanted. (If family members have to administer medications, this could be very difficult for some, impossible for others, and upsetting for everyone, including the patient, your parent.)

So, make sure that any home hospice care company or organization you contact can tell you the answers to all of the questions above, and make sure that the answers you receive are exactly what you want to hear. If not, take your business elsewhere or plan to move your parent into a facility (nursing home or hospice). Though we cared for my parent at home—at her request—the answers to the questions above would be the main reason for my recommending that end-stage care take place in a hospice or other facility. It is not easy to take care of someone with a serious illness at home. Do not push yourself to do it if you do not have the insurance, money, medical and family support that will allow you to do it well. In a facility, you have what you need on-site, no further away than a call-button or yell down the hall. This won't make your parent's passing less difficult, but it may be what you and your family need to feel more comfortable during the process. So, know what you need and want, and make sure that whatever arrangement you select can accommodate it.

Because hospice care provides round-the-clock care (24/7 care) and attention for very ill patients, please make sure that you read the last tip, "Understanding Twenty-four-Seven Care (24/7)."

How To Handle Special Issues

- Preparing for a Hospital Stay

- Using Silver Alerts to Find a Parent Who Is Lost

TIP 21

Prepare, to Have a Good Hospital Stay

How to Improve Your Parent's Hospital Stay

The Problem

If your parent is showing pronounced symptoms of his illness, it is a requirement that you plan your hospital stay well. Often, people do not get what they want from their parent's hospital stay because of three things:

1. **Hospital.** They don't research local hospitals; they just go to the closest one or the one that is familiar from when they broke their arm two years before. They don't know whether there is a gerontology department in the hospital, or whether they have special doctors or areas in the hospital that handle Alzheimer's or other dementia patients (for example, perhaps there is a floor in the hospital that is better prepared to house a patient that has a tendency to wander or maybe one hospital has designated staff to sit at bedsides or in corridors to attend patients). They don't know whether the hospital did well on its accreditation or not. They may not even know whether or not their neighbors like the place, or if the neighbors do like it, then they may pay too much attention to that fact.

2. **Doctor.** They don't have the right doctor, one they can rely on to communicate with them and with the nursing staff in a way that will help. Instead, they stick with someone who will not talk to them in a way that they can understand, someone who doesn't answer or return their calls, someone who frankly isn't very interested in their parent's problem, someone who might be

     great at making the common cold bearable or handling next year's bout of flu, but who isn't the best choice for this patient at this time.

3. **Nursing Staff.** They don't talk directly to the nursing staff and let them know facts that could help the staff do their job better, like the fact that the parent has a tendency to wander, or cannot sleep without a light, or gets agitated in unfamiliar places, or cannot feed himself. The nursing staff members are the people who will interact the most with your parent. The doctor will be there for the surgery or other procedure. The nurses will be there for that, as well as for everything else before, during, and after it. They are the day-to-day caretakers when it comes to hospitals and they can only be as good as the information you give them and the arrangements the doctor makes with them.

Not only should you be careful not to turn a good hospital staff into a not so good staff through your lack of communication, but also you need to be able to recognize when you and your parent need a change. Do not let loyalty to a facility, a location, or a person thwart your ability to get your parent the best care possible. Pick a hospital that is appropriate for your parent, not your child, not your broken arm. Pick a doctor who knows how to act as a positive connection between you and the nursing staff.

My Saga

When I walked into a local hospital, I found my very modest and dignified mother perched on the side of her bed, her hospital gown askew. She was unaware of my presence, almost oblivious to it, in fact. She was unable to feed herself, though she made the attempt, repeatedly trying to grasp a bit of food in her hand and get it up to her mouth. Each time failing. Her food tray sat on the table beside her bed, full, almost untouched. I was upset. Here she was alone, trying unsuccessfully to feed herself, and no one was anywhere around. The railing on her bed was down and she could have easily slipped off the side. (My mother had been a nurse, an R.N., she had taken care of patients who were in a similar condition, and I was very aware of how a patient should be looked after. This wasn't it.) It took everything in me not to rip her door off the hinges and clobber the staff with it. (Please remember that this was a passing feeling, not an act. *Keep such passing moments of anger and frustration in the feeling zone. Do not act on them.*) This moment occurred after almost a week of not hearing back from the doctor who had admitted my mom after an office visit. The doctor insisted that day that I should take my mom to the hospital right away. The doctor said she would let them know we were coming, and she would be over shortly to confer with me. Instead, it had been a week since my mother entered the hospital, with no calls from the doctor, no messages left for me with the nursing staff, nothing but silence and my mom sitting in the hospital room. I didn't understand why the doctor had admitted her. I didn't know what was supposed to be happening or what I should be looking out for or planning for. I didn't know what medications my mom was on and why. I didn't know what to tell my siblings, who were strewn all over the country at the time. As you can imagine, my siblings and I were not only unhappy but frightened and confused by the situation. Suffice it to say we were not anxious to return to either that doctor or that hospital. They probably were not anxious to have us back, either, because we spent much of our time trying to get answers out of them that they didn't have. The doctor was the key, and we couldn't find the key.

A Solution

What is the moral of the story here? You need to do some preparation before you go to a hospital. You need to make sure that both the hospital and the doctor are the right ones and you need to communicate with the nursing staff to ensure that they remain that way.

1. **Hospital.** Check out hospital facilities before you need to go there. Read those city magazines that run annual articles like "these are the best hospitals in the city." Baltimore, Boston, Chicago, Seattle, and San Francisco, all have these magazines. Your city may too. Find out, buy them, and read them.
2. **Doctor.** When it comes to doctors, you need to know two basic things: 1.) is the doctor connected to the hospital that you found in your research and liked and 2.) will you be confident and comfortable entrusting your health and possibly your life to this particular doctor.

    First, make sure that the doctor can take care of you at that facility. Why do I say that? I say it because doctors can only work in hospitals where they have privileges. Usually, doctors are associated with several hospitals in an area, and only under special circumstances may they obtain guest privileges in hospitals to which they are not already formally attached. So, if you go to a hospital where your doctor does not have privileges, another doctor will likely have to treat your parent or your doctor will have to see whether or not other arrangements will be allowed. Save time, save frustration, and pick a doctor that is already associated with the hospital you want to go to. Second, know your doctor. Know what he or she means by "I will contact you." Know how to reach the doctor—not only at the office, but also through his or her emergency service—and if possible, have the name of an alternative physician whom your doctor trusts and who will be on duty if and when your doctor is not. And if this doctor doesn't work out, don't be afraid to go to the next doctor, the one after that one, and so on until you find one that suits you and your parent.

Now that you think you know which doctor you want to see, you need to find out the details that will let you know you made the right choice. You need to know that you can reach him or her when you need to. You need to feel at ease with him or her and the staff at the office, and yes, personality counts here. Why would you spend your time and hard-earned money on someone you find rude, or annoying, or snobby? And always use the five-year-old test: Do you feel that you could leave a five-year-old that you loved in his or her care or the care of one of his or her staff members without worry? If not, that's a clue that this is not the place for you. You and your parent are just as precious as that five-year-old, remember that and make sure that you take care of yourselves.

So, call the doctor's office, ask his staff whether or not he is taking on new patients. If he is, make an appointment, and go. When you go, look at the office, notice the relaxation or tension of the staff, look at the cleanliness of the facility, notice how long you wait after the appointed time. Look and listen. Don't ask a ton of questions—though you should always ask about what you want to know—just be observant.

For that first appointment, ask the office staff whether they have a website where you can download, print, and fill out the mounds of paperwork every new patient is required to submit. If not, perhaps, if there is enough time before the appointment, they can mail it to you to fill out. That way, you can fill it out a little at a time, in the comfort of your home, without having to balance a clipboard on your knee as you keep an eye out for your parent and try to remember which surgery he had three years ago. Your parent will also be more relaxed and can probably help you fill in all those blanks on the form. (*I stress not having to attend to your parent while you prepare this paperwork because sometimes we forget how challenging it can be taking a parent out, particularly if your parent is at a later stage in his illness. He might be incontinent and need to be taken to a restroom right away. He may talk aloud disturbing the doctor's other patients, or attempt to leave the office and wander about if you aren't watching him every moment. None of this is too big a deal or is insurmountable, but it helps if you can just sit still for 15 minutes, undisturbed and pay attention to those forms.)*

Another suggestion, if you have a more flexible schedule and getting time off from work or other obligations to take your parent to the doctor's is not an issue, consider dropping by the office yourself to fill out the forms. The benefit of going alone that first time is that if the office is really horrible to get to, if the building has narrow corridors that make it difficult to maneuver a wheelchair in and out, if it just doesn't look like it should, or it has an office staff more suitable to a construction site than a place where people go to be helped and healed, you can turn around on your heels, go back to your car, and call them from your cell phone to cancel the appointment, then forget you ever heard about them. If this happens, then once again, go back to your research and find another doctor. Repeat as often as necessary. When both your mind and your gut are satisfied, then you will know you have made the best choice and can relax and begin making this new doctor, *your* doctor.

3. **Nursing Staff.** You need to make special arrangements whenever your parent is in a hospital. Alert your doctor to this concern in case he forgets. Talk to the nursing staff. Make sure your parent is in a special Alzheimer's or other dementia care area or that the staff is aware of his condition and any potential issues. Once I talked to the staff and explained the problem with my mom, I was able to get certain concerns handled. You and the nurses must be clear about how much and when they are going to sedate your parent. You must request that a nursing aide is with your parent twenty-four-hours a day, seven-days a week (24/7)—and yes, it will cost you more money. If your parent needs to be fed and cannot feed himself, the staff needs to be told this. After I requested these three things (only light sedation—if any, a nursing aide and feeding assistance), I slept well for the first time in a couple of days. Do not assume the nursing staff will figure it out for themselves. Your parent has probably learned how to get along without using many words. Your parent may be embarrassed to tell them or might not be *able* to form the words to tell them that he needs help with something. Do not wait to request help until your parent has gone without food for several meals in a row because

the staff assumes your parent can feed himself and just doesn't want what's on the food tray. The nurse may not realize that an orderly is picking up a full tray that your parent hasn't eaten. (It is not that unusual for patients to shun hospital food; it happens often.) Do not wait until your parent is attempting to join the doctors in their rounds while a less-than-sensitive nurse giggles, and you reach for the aspirin. Though thankfully this was not the case with my mother, don't wait until your parent is—as the character Harry Sanborn is in Nancy Meyers's movie *Something's Gotta Give*[20]—stumbling around the hall half-clad.

Your Solution

Make a Plan for Your Parent's Hospital Stay:

- **Get a nursing assistant to sit with your parent.**

  - It prevents wandering and gives your parent an immediate point of attention. It needs to be a 24/7 watch.

- **Make a list of things the nursing staff needs to know about your parent:**

  - There is a big difference between keeping your parent out of the room next door and making sure he is not in the gift shop or walking out in the parking lot to find a car that's not there. Make sure staff know if this is a possibility.

  - Does your parent wander?

  - Where and for how long?

  - How far is he likely to roam?

---

20 "Something's Gotta Give," 2003 film, Nancy Myers, writer and director, IMDb.com, accessed August 1, 2017, http://www.imdb.com/title/tt0337741/ .

- **Call and ask:**

  o **Do they have clergy or lay religious representatives who can visit your loved one, and how are they contacted? Must you be there to assist in interpreting your parent's situation or need to the clergy, or can they simply sit with your parent for a moment in your absence?**

    A pastor visited my mom while she was in a hospital once and he actually ended up giving me a great deal of comfort.

  o **Are there other visitors like assistance or therapy dogs that come in with handlers and allow the patient to pet them?**

    On the night that therapy dogs visited my mom in that same hospital, she ate for the first time that day. It was only half a cup of applesauce, but I felt relieved, and she looked better for the warm but cold-nosed company.

  o **Additional inquiries you might make to hospital staff:**

    If it's the holidays, are there Christmas carolers? Are there special meals for Hanukkah, Ramadan, or other religious holidays? All holidays can be celebrated at a hospital. Just take the time to plan. Contact the staff; see what's available. It may be the first time they have had this request, but that does not indicate a lack of caring or the possibility that next year someone else of your faith might not need to arrange something special, because it will have already been added to the menu, thanks to you.

Calming Advice

Try to remember that nurses, doctors, orderlies, and so forth, though professional medical workers, are also human beings. No, they shouldn't giggle when your parent wants to join the doctors on their rounds, or your parent does something else odd. They should be trained better than that. Sometimes, however, you must remember that it's their way of laughing *with* your parent, not *at* them. I'm not saying that you should tolerate rude or disrespectful behavior toward your parent. I am saying that if you get a grip on yourself and sometimes try to see the funny in it, you'll last longer. If you get irate every time something happens, your tread will wear out long before this road ends. If you warn the hospital and make arrangements for special care ahead of time, some of these incidents can be avoided.

Start using the information in the tip "Take Care of Yourself and Your Life," so that you'll be healthy while this is going on.

TIP 22

Use Silver Alerts to Help Find Your Parent When Lost

How to Use Silver Alerts to Help Locate Your Missing Parent

Understand What a Silver Alert? Is[21]

You have probably heard of Amber Alerts for missing children. Silver Alerts are for missing persons in the United States, (particularly senior citizens) suffering from dementia (Alzheimer's and other types of dementia), or another mental disability, illness, or condition. They are available in many, though not all, states. (See this link: https://en.wikipedia.org/wiki/Silver_Alert.)

Silver Alerts are announced on TV and radio stations, posted on electronic boards along highways, and sent as notifications for those accessing emergency information on smartphones. Whether Silver Alerts are formally available in your area or not, call the police (**dial 911**) if your parent goes missing, whether he is on foot, driving a car, or is a passenger in a car.

Prepare to Use Silver Alerts

Before you need Silver Alerts, learn about Silver Alerts. Go to your home computer and access your state police website, visit your local library and specifically ask for

---

21 "Silver Alert," Wikipedia, accessed November 29, 2016, https://en.wikipedia.org/wiki/Silver_Alert .

help, or stop by your local police station, if you feel comfortable going there. You need to know the following:

1. **Are Silver Alerts available in your community?**

2. **When and how do you use this service?**

   o **Who will a Silver Alert locate?**

      – For example, must the person be over sixty-five years of age or can they be younger than that if they have a mental illness?

      – Can anyone missing and over 65 be searched for under Silver Alerts or must there be a mental illness before this form of search can commence?

      – Do you need to have proof that the missing person was officially diagnosed with dementia (Alzheimer's, etc.) or another mental illness?

   o **How long must the person be missing before you can call?**

   o **Exactly how do you access and use the service? Call 911?** Is there an additional phone number to use in your jurisdiction?

   o **Exactly what information does the officer need from you if and when you do call?**

   o **Can a photo of the missing person somehow be uploaded to the police department from your home computer,** not only to save you a trip to the police station, but also to ensure that you are at home if the person returns?

3. **How can you, your friends, and neighbors track or monitor Silver Alerts?**

4. **Is there anything the community can do to make Silver Alerts either more useful or less necessary?**

Learn to Request a Silver Alert

If your parent isn't home and you are worried, or your parent has gone missing from around the home and you are afraid he may have wandered off, a Silver Alert might help you. **Always report your parent's absence immediately**—and it should be as soon as you've determined your parent is gone. It is surprising how far someone can go on foot or in a car in a short amount of time, so time is of the essence. **Call 911. Request a Silver Alert. If the dispatcher is unfamiliar with the term, tell him it's like an Amber Alert, only for seniors with dementia or other mental illness.** The detailed steps are below:

1. As soon as you suspect that your parent has gone missing, immediately contact your local police department by dialing 911.
2. Tell the police that you want to request a Silver Alert. Explain that your parent has dementia. Tell them whether your parent is in a car (and have the make, model, and license number handy, if possible), or if your parent was on foot (give them a direction he was headed). If you don't know for sure, give them the direction your parent tended to travel. For example, perhaps he usually left the house and walked to the left when he went to the park on the corner. Please make sure, however, that you tell the police that you do not know for sure whether your parent took that route, but rather that it was just his habit. That way the police will know how to use the information you have given them, and you may save precious time.
3. Quickly re-check the usual places your parent goes around the home.
4. Check the surrounding area.
5. Phone any neighbors, relatives, or even local businesses (if you live near them) who might have seen your parent walking, or offered your parent a ride to the store, not realizing the situation and his dementia issues. Get them looking too.

Learn to Respond to a Silver Alert

Do not just use the Silver Alert system to help yourself; make sure it's effective for everyone by always being on the alert for Silver Alerts and responding. Here are some steps to help you:

1. Set your smartphone to receive emergency alerts. Usually both Silver Alerts and Amber Alerts will be included.

2. Your phone will display notification messages with, for example, the license plate and description of a car carrying or being driven by a person with dementia or another mental illness who may need assistance. These notices are often also displayed on electronic boards along the highway.

3. If you spot the vehicle in question, try to notice one or two things: the highway sign, route number, or mile marker, for example, and the time. Notice which direction the vehicle was headed (that is, whether the vehicle was on your side of the road or headed in the opposite direction).

4. Do not stop on the highway or road to alert the police that you have seen a person or vehicle listed in a Silver Alert; it may not be safe to do so. For instance, it might be dangerous to pull off a highway to the uneven pavement or gravel on the side of the road, and even more dangerous to try to go from a stop to highway-level speeds in time to move back into traffic. Instead, **as soon as safe and appropriate, go to a well-lit store parking lot or some other safe location, park your car, and call the local police with the information by dialing 911. Let the operator know immediately that you are responding to a Silver Alert.**

One day, I observed a man pacing back and forth on the side of a local road. He walked for a while in one direction and then turned and headed back in the other direction. He seemed to want to cross the road, but was confused about the traffic lights. When all of the cars were stopped, he seemed afraid to move. I pulled over in the shopping center and called the police. I told them what road he was on and the businesses he was near, described him, and told them my concern. I stayed put at the shopping center until I saw the police squad car approaching the area, slowing down, and looking for the man. It made me feel much better.

Please Both Use and Respond to Silver Alerts

I will never know what the situation was with that man—maybe he ran away from home, maybe he didn't read English well and was confused by the signs, maybe he'd had too much to drink, maybe he had undiagnosed dementia—but I slept better knowing he wasn't lost in the woods that were near him and that he got somewhere safe.

Please do the same for Amber Alerts. The more eyes out there, the easier it will be for the police to find the ones we love and get them home to us.

How To Assist With Estate Preparations, Whether Your Parent Has A Lot Or Not

- Family Valuables and Family Relationships

- Your Parent's Will

- Planning Funerals and Memorials

TIP 23

Help Your Parent Navigate Deciding "Who Gets What" and Maintain Family Valuables and Relationships

How to Maintain Family Valuables and Relationships

Know What Your Parent Needs to Think about When It Comes to Distributing Valuables

This tip will help you to help your parent get ready to prepare his will. It is always so much better and easier to think about the ramifications of this issue, dividing property among family members, and avoid family squabbles, then it is to try to repair the damage to family relationships that some of these decisions often create.

Understand Who Gets Your Parent's Property and Other Items

Probably one of the most delicate subjects is the idea of who gets what property or items when your parent is gone. Not only is it a delicate subject, but it is one that must be decided before he draws up his will.

Parents do not like to think about the "who gets what when I'm gone" topic, and we don't want to push them to talk about it, but somebody's got to say something about it, or it's going to be a mess. Why a mess? All of you children may want the same bowl that mom served you oatmeal in when you were young. Your brother may assume that he's going to get the weekend cabin and start stocking it with his belongings and his friends, so that you are virtually locked out of using it. Things may suddenly start to disappear out of the house when one or another sibling visits and takes something he or she is "sure mom wants me to have." I know of people whose parents are so averse to discussing these issues that they are planning to leave it to the siblings to duke it out after they are gone. Let us try for something a bit more civilized and friendly than that. I suggest that you insist that your parent (either alone or with his spouse, if the other parent is still living), address the issue now. If that fails, go the uncivilized route—with one twist. You and your siblings duke it out while your parent(s) is/are still alive, well, and have to listen to it. I guarantee this will get them to voice some opinions and divide their property in some manner. It will not be perfect. People may not talk this holiday season, but it will be done, and you will thank me after your parents are gone, and you are not still trading barbs about who got their used Pyrex®.

If your parent is very ill, it should go without saying that you had better not be worrying about who the heck gets the bowl with the peacock on it. Focus on your parent and sort out the material issues later, even if you have to arm wrestle your siblings for the bowl.

Understand Who Gets Your Parent's Home

If your parent's home is something you or a sibling may want, make it known *now*. Also, if at all possible, make sure your parent decides who gets the home and informs all of the children of his decision. It might also be a good idea if your parent could explain *why* he made his decision that way. For example, if say one of the two children will inherit the house and the other will not, the child who will not inherit might feel slighted, *for the rest of his life.* Perhaps your parent could reconsider leaving the house to both of you kids. You kids could enjoy it together somehow or at least have that option. If that is out of the question, then wouldn't it be better for the siblings to know that the reason dad left the house to one sister, let's call her Kate, is that Kate is an artist, who could use the extra space for her studio, and since the place has a low mortgage she can afford to take a chance on the art she loves? Wouldn't it be even better if dad also said that he didn't leave the house to Stella, the other sibling, because he knew she loved the idea of living abroad and wanted her to feel free to have that adventure now—while she was still free of the job and family responsibilities that can sometimes make such adventures more difficult or impossible—rather than change her plans because she has inherited (and become saddled with) the old house? (As we all know, what is a blessing to one person can be a curse to another.) That's much better than Stella thinking dad was overlooking her again, or Kate thinking dad thought she was ridiculous for pinning her hopes on an artistic career and left her the house because he felt sorry for her (not proud of her).

Remember, if your parent has a vacation home, then he needs to make decisions about that as well.

Understand Your Parent's Home's Mortgage

If you or a sibling live in your parent's home and you may want to stay there, make sure you understand your parent's mortgage situation and check out inheritance law in your state. If there is a mortgage, can you assume it? If the mortgage is paid, can you afford the property taxes? Do inheritance laws require that you pay anything when the property is given to you? Such knowledge may be, for instance, the difference between your continuing to live in your parent's home for a year (or longer) after he passes away, simply paying his current mortgage, and your having to rush out and formally qualify for a mortgage of your own and purchase the house in order to have a roof over your head, while you're still reeling from several months or years of caretaking.

Consider Two Ways to Handle Gifting Other Items Your Parent Wishes to Leave to You and Your Siblings

Have each sibling e-mail a list of the things that mean the most to him, then there are two ways it can go from there. They can draw straws or your parent can distribute parent-selected items by appointment.

Draw Straws for Who Gets What

If there's no contest for an item and your parent is willing, then designate it for that person. If there is more than one person who wants an item, let them draw straws. Perhaps the person who lost will get his or her choice item in the next round. Or come up with a rule so that you make sure each sibling gets at least one item he or she desires and will love and enjoy.

Distribute Parent-Selected Items by Appointment

Another way to handle it is to give each person an appointment to come see his parent, and the parent gives that person what he has set aside for him or her. So, if you like the bowl with the peacock on it, perhaps you can drop hints to your mom (actually telling your parent straight out is best, when possible), and then your mom can just give it to you straightaway, and you do not have to worry about not receiving it later. Of course, this may mean that your parent is parting with belongings sometimes years before he needs to, so please consider this as an alternative only when there are one or two keepsakes to be gifted and not an entire household.

Consider These Ways Handle Items Your Parent Wishes to Leave to Outsiders—or Friends or Relatives You Just Don't Know Yet

Other Relatives

Your parent should also state whether relatives outside the immediate family are going to be given anything. There is nothing worse than some cousin from Florida, whom you barely know, taking the one item that meant the most to you, just because you had no idea of your parent's plans to gift the item outside of the immediate family, and your parent didn't realize how you felt. Make your voice heard now, so that you do not have to hold your peace for the next twenty family holiday dinners.

Charity

Your parent should also indicate whether funds or property (cars, art, books, etc.) will be given to charity. He should be sure to contact the charitable giving office of the organization in question to ensure that he knows how to properly designate the organization in his will. There are numerous charitable organizations out there and some of them have similar names. Make sure that gifts and donations reach the correct organization.

Dividing property and keepsakes beforehand and informing everyone of all decisions is, and always will be, the best thing to do. After all you are going through, surprises at the end are *not* what you need. You, especially if you are the child who will be handling power of attorney responsibilities (i.e., you will be making decisions for your parent and dealing with your siblings all along), need assurance that things will be well taken care of and peaceful at the end.

TIP 24

Ensure Your Parent Has a Will

How to Deal with Your Parent's Will (Last Will and Testament)

Caveat (Warning)

am not an attorney, nor am I an expert on wills. Get an attorney and consult him or her for any and all issues concerning wills (or powers of attorney, or such things as Living Trusts and Living Wills, etc., which your parent may also need to consider). These are general suggestions based on what I witnessed during my father's and mother's passing.

Ensure There Is a Will

Make sure that your parent has a will. No matter how much or how little money your parent has, he needs to have a will, especially if his spouse is no longer living. Your parent's will indicates what he wants to happen to the money he scrimped and saved over the years. Will it go to charity? To the kids? To the grandkids? A will designates what your parent wants to have happen to his property after he is gone. Whatever it is, he can make sure his family knows his wishes by indicating them in a will. These are decisions that affect families for years to come, financially, and also emotionally, in happy or hurt feelings. Please give your parent the chance to put in place the best choices that he can. My understanding is that your parent needs to be, to quote the old movies, "of sound mind" to draw up a will. Therefore, make sure that this tip is followed sooner rather than later. So, find out whether or not your parent has a will.

If not, then find an attorney, take your parent, and have a will drawn up. If you have no idea where to start looking to find an attorney, try using your computer again. Go to FindLaw.com—which I have used, but not for my mom's will or power of attorney since she already had her own attorney. Look up "Estate Attorney" or if you prefer try "Elder Care Attorney" or "Elder Law," and see whether that helps you at least start your search for the correct professional to assist you. There is also the National Academy of Elder Law Attorneys (http://www.naela.org/), which might be worth a look while you are seeking an attorney for your parent. (You and your parent might also be helped by the many eldercare-related articles available on the FindLaw.com website, or the articles available on the Legalzoom.com website.)

Why Ensure There Is a Will, Won't the State Handle It Anyway?

Won't the law indicate who gets things anyway? Yes, if you don't have a will, a judge will say, "Okay, this is [fill in the state name], and according to our laws, the surviving spouse gets it first, your parent's children get it next, and so forth." The list may vary slightly from state to state, but that's basically it. This division of property may suit your parent—or it may not. There are all sorts of relationships, divisions, and issues within families, and if they're going to come out, they are going to come out when property needs to be divided. If your parent leaves a will, however, how his property is divided becomes his choice—at least to a certain extent and within reason. Therefore, make sure that your parent has a will. Period.

Without a will, especially if there is no surviving parent, everything from your parent's house to his bank accounts may be unavailable until your case comes up in probate court, which can sometimes take two years, or some other legal procedure is endured. You may not have two years to wait before you need whatever items your parent has left—cash, cars, houses, furniture, stocks, bonds, and so forth.

Include Arrangements for Pets and Assistance or Service Animals So They Are Not Abandoned

Whether we call them pets, companion animals, assistance animals, or service animals, they take care of us. When your parent is preparing his will, make sure that along with his home, his valuables, things he wishes to leave to his children, he also remembers to include arrangements for any animals he has. All animals need to be left to someone who will care for them, not dumped on someone who might not take the best care of them, and not abandoned on the street. Most animals cannot find enough food on their own, may get injured, may bite or injure a person or another animal, and will likely be picked up by animal control and euthanized. Make sure your parent's pets and service animals have better options.

TIP 25

Plan Some Aspects of Funeral or Memorial Services Ahead of Time

How to Make Final Arrangements

This is a delicate subject, but it's one that I need to discuss with you: final arrangements. Please don't be so upset that you leave it until you are heartbroken over the death of your parent and then still have to manage putting together a proper funeral service while you deal with relatives, caterers, florists, and all of the other individuals who are as necessary for endings as they are for beginnings.

Yes, the pressure will be on, because you may be the only person who remembers what hymns bring your parent solace, knows what religious verses or words comfort him, and understands what faith elements would mean something to him. So now or soon, before that pressure is on consider these things. Think about all of these parts of the funeral or memorial service ahead of time, while it's still peaceful, and try some of the suggestions in this tip to make it easier.

If Your Parent Will Discuss Final Arrangements

If your parent is the kind of person who would honestly prefer to have a say-so in these plans, then ask his opinion when he is well, and you can both laugh and joke through some of this information. Just ask your parent to jot down his preferences and stuff the sheet of paper in the folder with the will and power of attorney for later.

If Your Parent Won't Discuss Final Arrangements

If your parent wouldn't want to even hear about such arrangements, then be subtler. If you watch religious programming together, ask whether he likes the selection being sung—or what his favorite hymn was as a child. Ask whether he enjoyed the readings in church last week, and if not, what verses or quotes he does like. Sit with your parent and look through the family photo album, if there is one. Ask what his favorite picture of himself is or which one he prefers of the whole family. If a spouse passed away first, gently ask your parent whether he has plans to be buried with that spouse or elsewhere, or whether he wants to be taken back home to grandpa's place.

What You Can Do and What You Can't Do

Some issues require word from a religious or civic authority. For example, can you use cremation or must you have a burial? Can your mom be buried in that special cemetery (a cemetery of a different faith, a veteran's cemetery, etc.) with your dad, or do restrictions apply? You need to find out about these issues as soon as you can, so that adjustments and appropriate arrangements can be made.

When you start, *first* seek out this information from a religious authority you trust (be careful here), a relative you trust who's had to make these arrangements before (be careful here too), on the Internet, or at a library. *Only then* should you visit your religious authority with your plan. Why search out information first? Because sometimes, at this most vulnerable time, people who are uninvolved in your suffering may say things to you that upset you. They may not mean to, but they will. They are going to be rushing or in the middle of other things and unable or uninformed of the need to focus on you gently. If you are told "no" to whatever you are proposing, it will be less of a shock if you found out ahead of time that "no" was a definite possibility. You will also know that "yes" is also a definite possibility and that there are places that can and will say "yes" to you and your plans. So instead of being defeated, you will know to keep trying at another location. For example, if someone says that you cannot cremate and brusquely walks away, don't be upset or offended. You know that you looked up a noted authority in your religion online, and that person said something different. Okay, so call the next house of worship, or a central information office for your faith and ask again until you get the information you need. In addition, you still have time to suggest the inclusion of other rites and traditions, rather than the one originally proposed, and you have the time to make whatever arrangements are necessary with those who will officiate or participate. Just remember to always verify any of these kinds of issues with more than one official, and at more than one location, if possible. Going back to the example above, I recently heard on a religious news show that for Roman Catholics you can seek cremation, but you cannot fling the ashes, for instance, into a lake. If you heard this show or if you just read this passage, the smart thing to do would be to contact your church or the nearest diocese and ask about the ruling. That way, you can confirm whether what I just wrote is true or false and figure out how it will affect your plans.

For Proprieties' Sake

Most houses of worship, in most faith communities have a group of people that run things. They are the ones that show up every week for services. They help in the offices. They make sure the flowers are fresh. They answer the telephone. They are also usually the first people you will speak with when you make any arrangements for your parent. Sometimes they're going to be helpful. Sometimes they're going to make it difficult for you. (And yes, some will even act like they, themselves, own the place.) Maybe it's because they don't know you. Maybe it's because they don't see you there every week. Here's my advice: Let it go. Ask these pillars, these members that have been there forever, what's best. I guarantee that you won't have the exact ceremony that you or your parent want, but I also guarantee that you will probably have a funeral or memorial service that satisfies the powers that be and the various factions you will have to live with and deal with in the future, and maybe for rest of your life. Give them a chance to let you know about all of the unwritten traditions that will be missed (and talked about by those in attendance) if you don't include them. Give them a chance to let you know how to do it *right*. With any luck, your parent will have a sendoff that helps and heals everyone, and you will be welcome there even after your parent is gone, which is when you will really need them.

You want to make sure that you do the right thing by your parent. That can look very different from someone else's version of the right thing, and some people may or may not approve of your choices. You know your parent. Go with what you, your faith, and the people you respect know to be right. Confirm what you're unsure about, make sure your religious group is satisfied with your arrangements, and try not to drive yourself crazy here. That is my best advice.

PART 3

Yourself

How To Improve Day-To-Day Life For Yourself

- What If You Can't Be There with Your Parent or Guilt Anyone?

- Manage Caretaking Caretaking with Siblings and Other Relatives

- Take Care of Yourself and Your Life

TIP 26

Learn How to Thoughtfully Opt-Out of Hands-On Caretaking

How to *Not* Be There with Your Parent--Participate Whether You Can Be There or Not

If You Just Can't Be There, Deal with Your Feelings (Guilt)

Maybe it's because you work in a sunny world, three thousand miles away from your mom's winter wonderland, and you need to keep it that way for right now. Maybe it's because you never got along well with your dad, and neither of you can see that relationship improving at close quarters. Maybe it's because you're in the military, and it's hard to commute from Germany. Maybe you're in school, just had a baby, or just bought a new house in another state. The reasons for not being able to be there with mom or dad are numerous. The resulting feeling is often the same: guilt. Either you make yourself feel guilty, or someone else dumps it on you.

You feel guilty if you love them, guilty if you don't like them too much right now, or guilty for putting your family, your work, your schooling, your life at the top of the priority list and considering those things alongside your parent's needs. Don't. Yes, there are scary stories of nursing home abuse. Yes, there are family members and neighbors who will never think you've done enough. Yes, there will be moments when your parent feels lonely and calls you, upset or needing a pep talk, and you're just not there to hold his hand. But you are not the only one who can do those things for your parent. Assume that, whether it takes you a day or five weeks, you can locate professionals who will be there when you cannot. Assume there are doctors, registered nurses, practical nurses, nursing assistants, caregivers, nutritionists, exercise instructors, and home repair and service people who can do some of the things you cannot. They are paid well to be there when you can't, and many of them enjoy their work and will pass that joy on to your parent. They will be the patient voice when you cannot explain something for the tenth time. They can help your parent take his meals when you either can't get him to take a bite or can't be there wielding that knife and fork.

Decide What You Are Willing to Do

Can You Support Your On-Site Sibling?

If the On-Site Person Is Your Sibling (Or Another Close Relative of Your Parent's)
If the on-site person is your sibling (or another such relative), you may have a better situation than you think. First, if you do have a sibling on-site, be prepared to deal with some anger, guilt, frustration, and so forth, coming from his side. Second, figure out a way to deal with both your on-site sibling and with your parent anyway.

Strategy

- **Try to understand what it's like for your sibling.** That sibling who is there has lost a lot of his freedom, mobility, peace of mind, sleep, time, in other words, a chunk of his life dealing with your parent. That's why when you visit, he is in no mood for you to waltz in and take over. He is also not in the mood to hear that you're running out to the gym or have to meet your date, while his evening will consist of feeding your parent in the nursing home or doing the loads of laundry that someone with an illness can produce in one week. Your onsite sibling may gripe at you or try to guilt you or berate you. You need to be prepared for this, and you need a strategy for dealing with it. How do I know that these things are likely to happen? Because this is exactly how I felt as the on-site person for my mother when I called my sisters or brothers and asked for help or complained about my day with my mom.

- **Listening is great; suggestions that involve your doing something too—even from far away—are better.** Phones work in all states and most countries. Volunteer to make some of those preliminary calls to either locate a residence for your parent or locate services. Even a call to Sears about when they can come out to fix the refrigerator might help out your sibling. Yes, it's minor, but you just saved your sibling his lunch break on a Wednesday. Maybe that's the only good thing that happened to him that day. If it's practical, if you can do it from where you are, do it. Not all the time, but at least every now and then. Maybe you're better at talking to the cable guy. So, give him a call, and give your sibling a break.

Can You Give Some Support to Your Parent's Non-Family Member Caretaker or Some Monitoring of the Facility's Care?

If the On-Site Person Is a Caretaker Who Is Not Related to Your Parent

If the on-site person is a professional caretaker, you may have less to be concerned about regarding the family relationship dynamics, but more concerns about safety and right fit of your parent to the facility (if applicable), the care level, and the specific caretaker(s). In this case, focus on maintaining "eyes-on" contact with your parent, that caretaker(s), and with the facility.

Strategy

- **Make sure your parent is in the right kind of facility for him and that he is content there from the start.** First, read the Tip 18 on Care and a Housing/Living Situation, especially the information on Option 4, Facilities, to get more ideas on how to make this arrangement work for you and your parent. Next, go back and read Tip 16 about assessing your parent's care needs and Tip 17 about how to pay for your parent's care. Selecting a good place for your parent will give your parent the care he needs, and minimize both your concerns and the time and energy you have to put in into the situation.

- **Even if your relationship is strained, communicate—at least minimally—with your parent and be your parent's "detective" when you call**. As has been mentioned, cell phones allow face-to-face communication, even at very long distances. Call your parent, at least minimally. These face-to-face calls will allow you to look in your parent's eyes to see whether their eyes are cloudy from too much sedation, or circled and distressed looking from not enough sleep, which is a possible sign of a noisy facility, of the wrong roommate, or simply of living too long in a situation that is uncomfortable for any number of reasons. You will notice a fake smile versus a real one. You will notice whether his or her roommate's sounds in the background are okay and allowable or present too much noise, distraction, or concern for your parent to remain in that particular situation. You can even notice how your parent reacts when a nurse or other facility official enters the room.

- **Find a way to visit or have someone else visit the facility where your parent resides**. It's great to visit your parent regularly, if you get along with them. If you don't get along with them, it's normal not to visit or not to visit as often. Such arrangements are fine when things are going well: your parent is in a safe, clean, and appropriate facility; he is treated well; he appears well-adjusted and content. If, however, you notice anything that concerns you, someone needs to be able to go to the facility and handle it.

  - **You (or a Sibling) Visit** - You need to actually go to the facility, whether go to the facility means a conference call to its head administrator or a plane ride and a rental car. Go to that facility yourself as soon as possible or send somebody you trust who lives closer to the facility. Families come in all kinds. Perhaps, unfortunately, you don't like your parent. That doesn't matter. Though you may not like your parent, you also do not want to have to live with his having been hurt in that facility and your not doing something about it. Think of your parent as a stranger if it helps. Don't feel like you have to recreate the happy family you never were or pretend to be something you're not, if that is an issue, just go or send someone immediately.

Can You Appoint a Guardian to be On-Site for Your Parent?

If the On-Site Person Is a Non-Related Guardian You Designated to Assist Your Parent
A Guardian for your parent is similar to a guardian for a minor child. This person is someone you trust who will care for your parent's needs—medical, financial, etc., If your being there for your parent is truly something that you either cannot do or do not wish to do (and do not feel guilty for feeling this; some parents have earned your feeling this way about them), then please consider designating a guardian for your parent. This person might be an attorney, another professional, or someone else. The idea is that the guardian would be in your parent's location, able to monitor your parent's care, and also equipped to intervene in that care. If something should happen to your parent, the guardian would know what to do about it and how to do it. His or her job would be to protect and care for your parent from the point when the guardianship is established to your parent's death (or until another time that you designate—for example if you are out of the country for three years and will resume care after that time period). I am not an attorney and cannot give you any detailed information about such arrangements, but please consider a guardianship and contact your attorney or an eldercare attorney about it.

Strategy

- **Your Parent's Guardian Visits** - Another alternative, as mentioned earlier, is to designate a guardian for your parent. This guardian would monitor your parent's care and intervene in that care if something should happen to your parent or should it become clear that a different facility would better serve your parent. Please consider this method and ask an attorney (and the facility where your parent resides) how to best employ this method.

My Experience
I felt guilty too, even though I was on site with my mom. I also felt proud to be there as a real grown-up for the woman who had always been there for me, and for all of us in fact. I'm even happy to say that my mother thrived a lot from my care.

But—and here's the rub—I also ran myself down, got sick more than I have since I was a really little kid, and developed a vitamin deficiency from poor eating, rushed lunches, and too much of "what's going on with her" and not enough of "what's going on with me." I spent too much money and started too many conversations with "Let me tell you about my mom." I gave up trips and outfits I wanted and other people I needed. So, do what I say, not what I did—that is, do not do that. God put two people here—you and your parent—not just one. Assume he meant for you both to thrive, not just one of you. Assume your parent can tell when you're pushing yourself too hard for him and that it probably doesn't feel good for him to be on the receiving end of your guilt and discomfort. Assume that your parent wants the best for you—even the ones who have never said it. Take your first step as a parent to your parent and stand firm for yourself, and your parent, when it comes to what you can do and what you cannot do, and select the arrangements that suit both of you.

TIP 27

Figure Out Ways to Manage Caretaking with Siblings and Other Relatives

How to Deal with Siblings and Other Relatives Involved in Your Parent's Caretaking

One of the most difficult parts of dealing with a parent or loved one's illness is dealing with the people closest to them and to you: the other family members. It's usually easy enough for everyone to agree that "we must take care of mom and dad." You may have siblings who live near or far; however, or who have very different ideas about what "take care of" means. Therefore, you need to ask and not assume you know what family members' roles will and will not be. Families come in various configurations. Not everyone has siblings, and sisters in one family do the job of aunts or nieces in another. Oh, and men are indeed included. I have known several men who have taken very good, hands-on care of their parents.

Consider Everyone's Current Situation

When it comes to dealing with siblings and other relatives, it's important to consider not just your feelings right now, but the entire situation and what you can and cannot expect from it. Here are some things to consider:

- Where do your siblings live—close to your parent or far away?

- Do their jobs allow them a flexible schedule?

- Do they have young children or other responsibilities that need to be factored in when it comes to assisting with your parent?

Try Not to Dump All of the Heavy Lifting on the Single Members of the Family

Here is my prejudice: please, please do not assume that your single brother or sister is just sitting around waiting to do his or her share plus some of yours just because she does not have a husband or he does not have a wife and kids. Single at thirty-five, forty-five, and so forth, is not the same as single at twenty-one (and I know that life was not easy for everyone at that age, either). Your single sibling has a mortgage, significant people in his life, and all sorts of adult responsibilities, just like you. Also, he may already be inundated by people at work who say, "I can't stay late; I have kids," and leave him hanging with extra work, holiday shifts, and so forth, because people view them as carefree people with nothing to do Give single people a break. Take their lives seriously and share responsibility. Even that wild brother of yours who actually does lead that fantasy single life of partying all the time needs a break every now and then, and the rest of us are tired of taking up the slack for the people around us. Dumping the heavy lifting on the single members of the family can do almost as much harm to your family as a crisis your parent might experience. Therefore, be conscious of this issue.

(Note: Do not misunderstand me when I discuss parents [and others] leaving to care for children. Yes, parents need to go, and they should be able to go. Many parents are just beginning to receive permission—given by time off and/or understanding of the need for more flexible arrival and departure times—the privilege to be there for their kids. We don't want to interfere with that; we want to encourage that; however, we also want people to be aware that single people have people depending on them too.)

If you don't have any siblings, your choices may be easier or harder. You may not have anyone else to take up the slack or with whom you can commiserate. But you also don't have anyone else to argue with. Also, those siblings whom you think make that other person with the big family lucky may not be as eager to take up the slack or ease the pain as you think they are.

Talk First, Not Last If You Know That You and Your Siblings See Things Differently

If you know or suspect that you are going to receive unsolicited (and possibly unwanted) advice from your siblings (or other significant relatives), get ahead of the conversation and ask for their input upfront. Why should you do that? Because if they are interested in giving advice, sharing thoughts, etc., then you have given them the opportunity to do so, which is a good thing to do. You get points for asking them and possibly get some useful information. Some of your siblings (or other significant relatives) will be helped by contributing to a person they love, admire, or have always been fond of. No one will feel left out. In addition, no one gets to say, "I told you so," because you asked them and they either chose to give you a suggestion that you seriously considered or they chose to say nothing. Most importantly, no one will be left with the feeling of not caring enough, not being there enough, or of not being included in helping your parent to be comfortable now and go on his way, peacefully. All will be well, with no regrets and no "if only's" after the fact, after your parent has passed away, and someone is concerned about how they could have been there, or how they might have helped, but didn't have a chance to do so. Furthermore, I found that the more I solicited advice, the more the people who didn't really want to be involved felt comfortable leaving the driving to me, so to speak.

Sometimes despite your best efforts and intentions, you will receive comments from people who can't or won't be there—either for reasons you know and understand or for those you don't—who will then blame you for your choices for your parent or for their own absence. Just remember, you're doing everything you can to do the best job for your parent. It's their concern talking. Though it may not sound good, it comes from a good place. Soothe them if you can. Let them go if you have to. Most importantly, continue taking care of yourself.

Go Gently (As Gently as You Can) With People Who Do Not Help

If, after all of this assessment, no one comes through for you, that's where paid help can pick up the slack. Do not waste too many hours mourning the fact that you are not related to the Brady Bunch or whatever fictional family you loved as a kid. Just get out there and find yourself some nice people who will be only too glad to help where you cannot, be there when you are busy, and hold your parent's hand when you need to be absent, for a fee. And try not to hold this against your siblings. This is the stuff that ruins families forever. Your parent won't always be ill. Your parent also won't always be here, and you're going to need these people when it's over and the dust settles. Do not burn your bridges. Families are made up of all kinds. The person who cannot be there for you the way you want them to now, might be just the person you need when you break up with your husband or get fired from your job. So, try not to expect more from people than they are capable of giving. Remember, God gave them their gifts—if you believe in that sort of thing—and neither you nor they chose which ones they would receive and which things they would do well. Sitting and holding your parent's hand just may not be something your sibling will be able to offer and give. Try to leave it at that—at least after you pound the wall or slam the receiver down. Call back tomorrow, say something nice, and keep him in your life. You'll need a shoulder to lean on when times get harder. The best one might just be your sibling's.

TIP 28

Take Care of Yourself and Your Life

How to Worry about Your Own Life the Right Way

Why Worry About Your Own Life?

People have heart attacks over this stuff. People die before their parents over this stuff. Newspaper and magazine articles talk about how caretakers die sooner than their counterparts of the same age due to the excessive stress. Don't be one of those people.

Remember, you need to take care of the person who takes care of your parent. That's you. You're the bottom of the pyramid. If you go, so does everything and everyone else. The key is to see that you have your own pyramid as well. There are things that support you and things that will make you topple. What makes you topple? What makes you lose your balance? Figure out what topples you, and you can avoid a lot of the strain that turns caretakers into those who need care themselves. So, what are those supports at the bottom for you? Is it your job? Your friends? Your faith? Your relationship? Your hobbies? What are those things that, when times get stressful, pull you through? And if you don't have those things in your life, what would you like them to be? Figure out what those supports are for you, and you have the makings of a good life and one of the most important things in this book: a means to take care of yourself.

Figure Out What You Need and What You Don't Need

It can be difficult to figure out what you need and what you don't need. Here are some suggestions. Use these to get started and add your own:

- **Job**

  - You need a stable job (Exception: If your current job is causing stress and a change of job will alleviate your stress or other problems, rather than add to it.)

- **Faith**

  - You need something greater to believe in, confide in, go to when you're troubled; some call it faith, some call it other things. You don't need judgment, damnation, aggravation, discouragement, or loneliness, though time alone is fine. (Exception: If what your parent is going through leads to your own journey, to your own spiritual or religious epiphany, self-exploration, or awakening—the kind that is not soul wrenchingly negative and destructive, but rather deeply cathartic and life-affirming.)

- **People**

  - You need people around you, real friends who can take you as you are, today (and love and care for you). You do not need negative people, busy-bodies, and onlookers. (Exception: If these onlookers see you falling apart and are capable of giving criticism constructively and positively and they can, and do, lend you a helping hand, then take it. That is a much-needed kind of interference, and whether they gripe a little along the way or not, you might want to consider keeping them on your side.)

What *Not* Figuring Out Your Needs Does

I Didn't Keep My Job Stable While My Mom Was Ill

Do not do what I did. I decided that in the midst of caretaking my mom I would take on a demanding job that required travel. Because of that obligation, I was three thousand miles away when things began to go wrong. Keep your nice, steady, boring job where they will let you flex your time and where they appreciate the fact that you are a good, reliable worker because they have known you at your best. Do not choose this time to try to make a good impression on strangers. Tell the Human Resources

Department what's going on, but keep your stories of woe out of the office. Offices are for making money, listening to coworkers' gossip, and eating donuts left on a desk. Try to only participate in the first activity. Avoid the other two. Remember, do not try to make coworkers into your support network, unless you are legitimate friends. What do I mean by "legitimate friends"? I mean people you already have an established friendship with outside of work, i.e., you go to each other's homes, you share at least occasional meals, you shop together or go to sports or cultural events together—you know, a real friendship. Even if you do have legitimate friends at work, still I would suggest you be careful about how much you share. Go to these people, of course, before you go to other co-workers, but remember, you don't always know their motives, even if they seem helpful, and you can't afford the fallout if ultimately, they're not. Be careful about how much you share. Even people we consider friends, people who mean us no harm, can make an odd comment at work that gets us written up, or gets people gossiping about us, or gets our boss wondering whether we're carrying our weight. Just be careful and keep your private life at home as much as possible.

I Didn't Go to a Church, Synagogue, Temple, or Mosque for Solace

I am a firm believer that God makes house calls. But you need not only heavenly support; you need human support. You need people who see the look on your face when you have talked to your parent who remembers that he knows you, but can no longer recall your name. You need someone who notices the twenty pounds you've lost or gained and does more than laugh about it with his friends. You need people who see your struggle and are there on the path with you, offering water and the occasional bandage. Remember, though, that people who are trying to follow or embrace a religion, faith, or spiritual connection are not perfect people. They probably will laugh, as that twenty-pound loss makes your pants fall off, or that twenty-pound gain makes your skirt squeeze the life out of you, so try not to be too judgmental or sensitive. I am not good at this, but I'm sure you'll be better at it. Give them a chance, though, and they will surprise you.

Also, don't forget religious or spiritual teachers and guides—priests, ministers, and so forth. You need people taking the journey of faith, but you need not only fellow travelers, but also a few trail guides, people who can assist you in finding the tools you need to both help your parent now and then let him go when the time comes.

I Didn't Join a Social Group

You need to have fun. You need to laugh more than you cry. That means you need friends, dates, and activities, or time with your spouse and children if you have them. If you're single do *not* delay dating, but be aware that you will be needy because of the situation and be careful to spread some of that neediness around, among your friends, rather than putting it all on that new someone or the one poor friend that you find time to see. If you're married, be careful not to wear your mate out with stories of your parent's problems, or with taking on more than you are truly able to handle. Be a person, not just a worker bee. Give yourself a break from adulthood. And you parents who are being slammed on both sides of the caretaking quotient, give yourselves a break from mom-hood and dad-hood. Play for a while. One hour out will not make you a bad parent—just the opposite.

Build a Life for Yourself, If You Don't Have Your Own Life Anymore,

This section is especially for those who somehow forgot their own lives in the middle of helping someone else with his or hers. If you don't have a life yet to maintain, focus on building it. Do not delay your own progress. Your parent needs the happiness that new family will give you, the shelter your new home may provide, and the income the increased schooling or new job may offer you. And your parent wants the best for you, so he needs to see you fulfilled, happy, and smiling—even the ones who don't show it. So, learn to be a good parent to yourself. This is important whether you're a twenty-two-year-old or a seventy-two-years-old, and don't let anyone tell you otherwise. You will need a life after your parent is gone.

Make Creating a Satisfying Life a Priority

- Date.

- Get married.

- Have children.

- Go to that school or college you've always wanted to attend—and that includes the seventy-two-year-olds among you.

- Change to that preferred job.

- Learn to bake a pie, or swim, or dance, or play volleyball, or snowboard, or build a robot, or rebuild an engine, or invent the next must-have-high-tech-make-lots-of-money-with-it gadget, or [fill in the blank] with whatever makes you feel as breathlessly excited as this sentence reads.

- Just do something you've always wanted to do.

While you are building your life, remember to filter any and all ideas through your own needs, beliefs, experiences, physical and mental health, and common sense—always common sense. What do I mean by common sense? Well, if you've been doing nothing but sitting in your cubicle working, taking care of your parent, and driving home, then you probably are not in the best physical shape. Therefore, do not run out and start lifting 50 lbs. weights tomorrow and tell someone that I told you to do it. That's what I mean by common sense.

Maintain the Life You Have, If You Have Been Able to Keep Some of Life's Pleasures Going

You were probably already undergoing stress in your everyday life: the commute to work, the job, the boss, the coworkers, the deadlines, the children, the play dates and homework, the spouse, the in-laws, and the former spouse, but you managed it. Now you've added caring for your parent. Whether you're a hands-on caretaker who has to figure out how to pay all the extra bills coming in, or the adult child who has to worry about mom or dad long distance, it's difficult, and it can wear you and your body out.

Once you figure out what supports you and establish your life, here's how to take care of that life and yourself.

Keep Things Going

- **Get a complete physical.**

  - If you're feeling less than great, don't assume you know what's wrong. Get a complete physical.

- ○ If your doctor doesn't already know, then tell him or her that you have become your parent's caretaker and are experiencing heightened levels of stress.

- ○ Tell him or her if your parent's dementia is related to any form of illness, such as heart disease or stroke. That might make you more susceptible to the same illness, meaning that it's something the doctor needs to keep an eye on, and it might also mean that this stressful time is a very likely time that a similar condition might become pronounced in you.

- ○ Pay attention to your doctor's recommendations as much as you pay attention to the things your parent needs.

- **Don't add more stress to your life.**

- ○ Don't switch to a more demanding job.

- ○ Don't move unless you must.

- ○ Don't buy expensive things that you can only afford to pay for if you work overtime.

- ○ Don't work overtime. You already have a second job, which is taking care of your parent.

- **Renew your faith.**

- ○ Read uplifting books, whether specifically about religion or not.

- ○ Find a quiet place to pray. For example, it could be a formal building or a garden.

- ○ Visit faith communities. Try various places if it has been a long time or you have no formal faith.

- ○ Consider joining or making regular attendance at an appropriate and comfortable faith community part of your routine.

- **Do multiple things that bring you solace.**

  o Write in a journal.

  o Re-read children's stories that comforted you when you were younger.

  o Watch TV programs that make you feel good. (I used to watch *Mr. Roger's Neighborhood* on TV whenever I was home with a very bad cold. It made me feel cared for to hear his kind and gentle voice, and the peacefulness of the show would lull me to a restful sleep, which is usually what I needed most of all. If that program doesn't do it for you, try *Anne of Green Gables*, or *Little House on the Prairie*, or an old movie like *His Girl Friday*. Or if that's too old and too old-fashioned for you, re-watch the *Star Wars, Jason Bourne, James Bond, Die Hard*, or *Sex and the City* movies or try re-runs of *How I Met Your Mother, Two-and-a-Half Men, Friends, Frasier, The Cosby Show*, or *I Love Lucy*.)[22]

  o Take a yoga or other exercise class; make it relaxing, not challenging.

  o Take up a sport you love that you haven't played in a long time, one that puts you in the moment and takes you out of your worrying thoughts (or start becoming a regular fan of your favorite sport on TV, learn about its history, and focus on your love of the game).

  o Sleep late on Saturdays.

  o Renew a hobby, hike, knit, sew, work on that old car, make jewelry, ride, play basketball, play cards, cycle, or do whatever activity you enjoy.

---

22 Television series "Mr. Roger's Neighborhood" (1968-2001), "Little House on the Prairie" (1974-1983), "How I Met Your Mother" (2005-2014), "Two-and-a-Half Men" (2003-2015), "Friends" (1994-2004), "Frasier" (1993 to 2004), "The Cosby Show" (1984-1992), "I Love Lucy" (1951-1957); television miniseries "Anne of Green Gables" (1985), films "His Girl Friday" (1940), and film series "Star Wars" (1977-present), "Jason Bourne" (2002-present), "James Bond" (1962-present), "Die Hard" (1988-present), and "Sex and the City" (2008 and 2010), IMDb.com, accessed August 1, 2017, http://www.imdb.com.

- **See your friends more—and see more friends.**

  - Make time for the movies.

  - Meet friends for a quick lunch if you can't devote an entire evening.

  - Listen to your friends' problems, and give your own a rest.

  - Learn to dump your frustrations on several friends. Don't overburden one friend, and your friends will never know you're dumping.

- **Eat better.**

  - Skip the drink if you tend to drink too much. Instead, treat yourself to that steak or seafood dinner that's a little more than you would normally spend, but is something you know you'll enjoy.

  - Or if you never drink, and you are safely at home, have half a glass of wine and slowly finish that Lean Cuisine® meal instead of gulping it down.

  - If you're married or have a family, sit down and eat. Don't graze over the kids' plates or go all out for your husband or your wife but eat a frozen pizza when he or she is working late (unless of course, like me, you love frozen pizza—in that case it's a treat).

- **Slow down.**

  - Eat deliberately and more slowly.

  - Drive more slowly. Your brain might be more tired and less focused. Give yourself the chance to react properly without adding more stress.

- **Ignore onlookers, and don't overachieve.**

  - Everyone always knows how to raise your children and how to care for your parents, especially if they aren't going to so much as say hello to them. Do not let these know-it-alls make you feel like whatever you are doing or contributing is insufficient. They're probably criticizing you while they watch their shows on TV.

○ Some people think it's easy to monitor someone else's bank account; deal with issues that arise in his mail; make doctor's appointments; take him to doctor's appointments; remember all his records, x-rays, and medications; earn the money that pays for all the home-care and home-maintenance help, all the doctor copays, all the prescription copays, all the heat, all the air conditioning, all the gasoline, all the debt, all the clothing for another adult, plus pay for your own adult household and life. They mistakenly think it's the same as taking care of a child. It's not. We all know enough to know that being the parent to a child isn't an easy job. I'm not quite sure why people think being a parent to your parent is.

How To Navigate Final Moments

- Navigating Tasks and Thoughts

  - Before Your Parent Passes Away

  - After Your Parent Passes Away

  - When You Start to Recall Your Experience

TIP 29

Prepare for that Day Before Your Parent Passes Away

How to Prepare for Your Parent's Passing Away

Whether you call it dying or passing away, it all means that your parent is leaving you, forever. This is such a primal moment. When that person who, for better or for worse, was your first source of comfort, protection, and love, the person who was your first teacher and guide, leaves you, words cannot describe it. Many very strong, very together and well-established people are amazed at the effect it has on them and on their lives for years to come. So, expect it to mean more than you think it will and to touch you more than an adult should properly let it. Let the feelings wash over you. Don't resist them. It will be much easier if you let it happen.

Have a Plan for Before and During the Funeral or Memorial Service

Make a plan for when the end comes. When your parent dies, have someone to call, someone to come by immediately, and someone to hold your hand the day of the funeral or memorial service. I went through my father's funeral alone, though I had sisters, and brothers, and relatives galore surrounding me, because I didn't reach out to people and let them know that I needed them. I went through my mother's funeral with someone to hold me and it made all the difference. It can make the difference for you too. This is not a time to stand alone, if you can help it.

Have a Plan for After the Funeral or Memorial Service

Also, think about what you will want and need to do, not just to handle guests that attended the services, but to comfort yourself afterward.

If you are a reader, pick out a book that you will either re-read every couple of years or never want to see again for the rest of your life. Check your mood, and you'll know which way to go with this one. Next, pick out comfy clothes, the kind of clothes that you could live in for weeks if you wanted to (and people wouldn't beg you to get up and take a shower). Sit in a chair, curl up in bed, and immerse yourself in another world. Get to know the ease of a summer breeze in 1800's New England, or a camping trip in the 1950's, wherever there is life, and fun, and hope, easily available on the next page. When all else fails, go to this new place and rest there for a while.

There may be lots of people around at first; take advantage of it. Life will get quiet soon enough. There will come a moment when your home will be very still, and you will realize just how empty all those hours are that you used to spend with your parent, and you will realize how empty those rooms are without the sound of your parent's voice echoing. So, enjoy the noise and endure the visitors who are doing the hard job of showing up and being there for you.

TIP 30

Keep Busy, But Go Gently After Your Parent Passes Away

How to Handle Things After Your Parent's Passes Away

You're still numb I know, but there are things you need to do, and the doing will keep you too busy to remember that you are sad and blue, too busy to be upset because you never found the perfect parting words to share with your parent, and too busy to be angry about the flowers someone didn't send, or the words someone said.

Keep Busy Doing Things You Need (and Want) to Do

1. **Close-Out Dealings Regarding the Funeral or Memorial Service**

    First, list what has to be done to close out any funeral or memorial service dealings. Do you still have a bill to settle? Did you pick up the CD that played at the meal after the service, the one with the montage of your mom, dad, and all of your family, or is it still sitting in an office at the funeral home or another location? They probably deal with a lot of people and have lots of such items they must keep track of. After all of the hours it took you to pull it together and how you felt when you saw it, you don't want to leave it behind and lose those precious memories. Stop by or make an appointment, whichever is appropriate, and get that CD. Did you purchase all of the special effects, like the blown-up portrait of your dad or the special cards that carried your mom's favorite poem? If not, go to the funeral home and order them now. Remember to thank them and recommend them to others.

2. **Keep Your Parent's Personal Affects or Belongings, for Now; Don't Give Anything Away, Yet**

Second, if you have the luxury of a place to keep your parent's belongings for the time being, then do not: go-through, sort, or throw-out anything; leave it for at least a month. A lot of people toss mom and dad's junk that's taking up so much room, trying to seem brave. They run through this necessary passage quickly. Unfortunately, they usually end up back at the Good Will drop-off, the neighbor's house, or the church rummage sale in tears looking for what they gave away. You will be ready to act soon enough. For now, a little junk won't hurt you and getting rid of it won't heal what's ailing you. Maybe you are trying to rush because you're afraid that you will want to put mom's robe around your shoulders and never take it off. Maybe you're concerned about your urge to wear dad's old watch every day, even though it doesn't keep time well anymore, and should have been replaced a few years ago. I know those feelings. Don't think tossing those things out quickly will get rid of those feelings. In fact, stop thinking there's anything wrong with those feelings. After sometime, stop, look, and pick a few mementos, then give yourself the freedom to keep them close to you. Wear the robe on Saturdays. Keep the watch on your bedside table, next to the digital clock that works well. Also, make sure that your siblings and the grandkids (or others that would be appropriate) have the same opportunity to keep a little part of your mom or dad.

3. **Be Gentle with Your Emotions; You Will Be Up and Down for a While**

Third, be aware that your nerves are going to be a bit discombobulated. You are not going to know some days whether you're going to laugh or cry. Be mindful of this fact and don't be either too surprised by it or too upset by it. Years ago, on a Facts of Life[23] sitcom episode, the character Mrs. Garrett, who played the house mother and life counselor to four young girls at a boarding school, talked to one of the girls, Natalie, about her father's death. Mrs. Garrett recounted her own father's death and how she thought she was fine with it until she went to the movies with some girlfriends to see Billy Wilder's movie,

---

23 "The Facts of Life," 1979-1988 TV series, IMDb.com, accessed July 31, 2017, http://www.imdb.com/title/tt0078610/releaseinfo?ref_=tt_ov_inf .

Some Like It Hot, with Tony Curtis, Jack Lemmon, and Marilyn Monroe. She retold how she laughed so hard and then she cried just as hard. She explained to Natalie how it's hard doing other things after losing someone. You're afraid you're forgetting them in that moment of laughter and it makes you feel awful, because you want to remember them forever. I had similar reactions after losing my mom. I would watch something that she would love, and laughing begin to turn to say something about it to her, then I would remember she wasn't there anymore and wonder how I could be watching and enjoying this show now that she was gone. It may not be rational, but it happens. That's why I'm cautioning you. Let it go. Your emotions are tired and raw. They're going to be up and down. Don't expect too much from yourself right now. Give it time.

4. **Make a Special Effort Not to Overreact; Take It Easy**

    Fourth, this is also not the time to press yourself to operate in environments that require diplomacy, tact, or gentility. You will think you're behaving in a reasonable manner, but you may not be. The people you're talking to will notice, because you are uncharacteristically going on a tirade for twenty minutes about people who park too far from the curb, or eat soy, or about something some politician said. Take it easy. Assume you may overreact and don't debate or consider anything more important than which cute puppy picture is the best, and go gently with that too.

5. **Stick to a Routine or Start a New Adventure; Know which Person You Are and Be That Person**

    Fifth, immerse yourself in work, in baseball, in movies, but not in stress. This is probably not the time for new relationships that you will lean on too heavily, new jobs that will strain your internal resources too much, deciding to invest your money, or deciding to move to another country. Of course, if these things are restful for you, if they're the things that calm you, then pursue them, but pursue them with care. If you are a start a new adventure person, set some guidelines for yourself. Try to make your adventure: 1.) something you've always wanted to do (not a new whim) and 2.) something you're prepared to do (not something requiring a new skill set or an unusual amount of effort). Be careful deciding that you'll move to Germany and so you'll need to master Spanish from beginners to advanced level in one year. That is an example of too much. Your brain is tired. Don't push it. An Eat Pray

Love[24] style journey may be just the way to go, but ease into it. (Remember, in both the film and the book, she relaxed, ate, and regained not only the body weight she had lost in her divorce grief, but also some of her bearings before she set off on the intense spiritual portion of her journey. She didn't show up and on day one and start meditating for hours a day. Keep that in mind.)

---

24 "Eat Pray Love," 2010 Film, directed by Ryan Murphy, written by Ryan Murphy and Jennifer Salt, based on a book by Elizabeth Gilbert, IMDb.com, accessed August 29, 2017, http://www.imdb.com/title/tt0879870/?ref_=nv_sr_1 .

Epilogue
From Beginning to End

How I Had Some Very Good Years

Frank Sinatra sang a song called, *It Was a Very Good Year*[25]. In it, he talks about starting from age seventeen, when he's kissing small-town girls on the village green, to when he is an old man drinking in everything life has to offer, including the dregs—that last, crummy, sediment-laden part that's left at the bottom of the barrel. That is the way life is. These last years with your parent are going to be rough. They are going to test you in ways you cannot imagine. No, it's not like going to war or being in a horrible accident, but it's pain nonetheless, and it's a kind of pain that many people can't see.

I guarantee, though, that with the pain will come some of the best gifts life has to offer. Being one of five children, I had years of being the only kid in the house with my mom. I had years of taking her to McDonald's* and sitting and watching the leaves change with the seasons. I had years of holding her hand and being able to do for *her* for a change. It may not sound like much written here, but I think you will find it is a lot. It gives meaning to it all and makes it all bearable. We had some very good years.

---

25   Frank Sinatra, "It was a Very Good Year," September of My Years album (Reprise Records, 1965, on LP), accessed July 31, 2017, https://en.wikipedia.org/wiki/September_of_My_Years .

After You Read This Book

After reading this book, I hope you found that it helped you to hear from someone else who knows what it is to deal with a parent who has dementia. I hope you found that you learned a few things that you can now use. I hope you also found that you were moved to share what you learned with your siblings, your spouse, your kids, friends your age who are taking the same journey you are, and those who will be on the same road soon.

If you found anything useful in this book, please give me a review and let me know. If you found that it brought up stories you want to share, please give me a review and tell me about them. Your honest and polite comments are welcome and encouraged. Please add them to my book's page on Amazon.com or to the publisher's website, Stewartpublishing.com.

Thank you.

Add Your Own Tips

———————————————————————————————————————

U se the "Your Tips" pages that follow. The tip sheets can hold your own thoughts and ideas. These might be things you hear or read about in an article. They can be the things that will get you through when the going gets tough. They may give you something to pass on to the next guy, the way I've passed this book on to you. I wish you the best of luck and happiness in your journey.

YOUR TIPS

YOUR TIPS

YOUR TIPS

YOUR TIPS

Bibliography

AARP (AARP.org). *Dementia Diagnosis*. 2016. http://healthtools.aarp.org/health/de-mentia-test-and-diagnosis-testing (accessed November 20, 2016).

—. *What is Alzheimer's Disease?* 2016. http://www.aarp.org/alzheimers_disease_what_is_alzheimers.asp (accessed November 20, 2016).

Administration on Aging (AoA) UnitedStates Department of Health and Human Services. Alzheimer's and Dementia. 2017. https://aoa.acl.gov/ (accessed April 7, 2017).

Alzheimer's Association (ALZ.org). Alzheimer's and Dementia. 2016. http://www.alz.org/dementia/ (accessed November 22, 2016).

—. *Clinical Trials, Alzheimer's Association TrialMatch®*. 2017. http://www.alz.org/research/clinical_trials/find_clinical_trials_trialmatch.asp (accessed July 21, 2017).

—. *Types of Dementia*. 2016. http://www.alz.org/dementia/types-of dementia.asp (accessed November 22, 2016).

—. *What is Alzheimer's?* 2016. http://www.alz.org/alzheimers_disease_what_is_alzheimers.asp (accessed November 20, 2016).

Alzheimer's Disease Education and Referral (ADEAR) Center, National Institute on Aging (NIA), National Institutes of Health (NIH). Alzheimer's and Dementia. 2017. https://www.nia.nih.gov/ alzheimers (accessed March 13, 2017).

—. *Alzheimer's Disease Fact Sheet.* 2017. https://www.nia.nih.gov/alzheimers/publication/alzheimers-disease-fact-sheet (accessed June 19, 2017).

—. Alzheimer's Disease Research Centers [ADC]. https://www.nia.nih.gov/alzheimers/alzheimers-disease-research-centers#statelist (accessed July 21, 2017).

American Automobile Association (AAA.com). *Senior Driving.* 2017. https://midatlantic.aaa.com/traffic-safety/senior-driving. (accessed April 3, 2017).

American Geriatrics Society (HealthinAging.org). Eldercare and Help for Caregivers. 2017. (accessed March 13, 2017).

American Heart Association (heart.org) and American Stroke Association (strokeassociation.org). *Together to End Stroke. Stroke Connection.* 2017. http://strokeconnection.strokeassociation. org/ (accessed March 13, 2017).

BrightFocus Foundation (BrightFocus.org). *Amyloid Plaques and Neurofibrillary Tangles.* 2017. http://www.brightfocus.org/alzheimers/infographic/amyloid-plaques-and-neurofibrillary-tangles (accessed July 27, 2017).

Cleveland Clinic (My.ClevelandClinic.org). *What is Dementia?* 2016. http://my.clevelandclinic.org/health/diseases_conditions/hic_Types_of_Dementia (accessed November 20, 2016).

Eldercare.gov. A service of the U.S. Administration on Aging (AoA). 2017. http://www.eldercare.gov/Eldercare.NET/Public/Index.aspx (accessed March 12-13, 2017).

Harvard Nurses' Health Study (NHS) (nurseshealthstudy.org/). *History, Harvard Nurses' Health Study.* 2017. http://nurseshealthstudy.org/about-nhs/history (accessed July 2017).

Health Reference Library. A service of Healthline Media (Healthline.com). Alzheimer's and Dementia. 2017. (accessed March 13, 2017).

—. *What Do You Want to Know About Dementia?* Written by Wendy Leonard, MPH, Published September 15, 2014, Medically Reviewed by Timothy J. Legg, Ph.D., CRNP, quoted in "Dementia Diagnosis," Health Encyclopedia, AARP. org, http://healthtools.aarp.org/health/dementia-test-and-diagnosis-testing, (accessed November 20, 2016).

IMDb (Internet Movie Database) (IMDb.com). 2017. A database of information related to movies, as well as the writers, directors, actors, producers, and other cast and crew members involved with them. http://www.imbd.com (accessed August 2017 and November 2017).

Krause, Lydia. *What is Mult-Infarct Dementia?* (healthline.com) Edited by College of Medicine on March 16, 2016 University of Illinois-Chicago. http://www.healthline.com/health/alzheimers-dementia/multi-infarct-dementia#Symptoms2 (accessed November 20, 2016).

Mayo Foundation for Medical Education and Research (MFMER) (MayoClinic. org). *Dementia-like Conditions That Can Be Reversed, Dementia: Symptoms and Causes.* 2017. http://www.mayoclinic.org/diseases-conditions/dementia/symptoms-causes/dxc-20198504 (accessed March 13, 2017).

—. *Dementia Overview.* 2016. http://www.mayoclinic.org/diseases-conditions/dementia/home/ovc-20198502 (accessed November 20, 2016).

Medicare/Medicaid (Medicare.gov). Long-term Care and Other Care Opportunities. 2017. https://www.medicare.gov/ (accessed March 13, 2017).

National Institute on Aging, National Institutes of Health (www.nia.nih.gov). Alzheimer's and Dementia. 2017. (accessed March 13, 2017).

Oxford University Press. Oxford (English) Living Dictionary (OxfordDictionary.com). 2017 (accessed August 29, 2017).

Scripps Networks Interactive, HGTV (HGTV.com). *Aging In Place Home Technologies.* 2017. http://www.hgtv.com/remodel/mechanical-systems/aging-in-place-home-technologies (accessed March 22, 2017).

Social Security Administration (ssa.gov). *Find Your Parent's Benefits*. 2017. https:// www.ssa.gov/ onlineservices (accessed March 20, 2017).

Virginia Division of the Aging. *Alternatives to Guardianship*. 2017. http://www.vda.vir-ginia.gov/ (accessed March 20, 2017).

Wikipedia.org. Alzheimer's and Dementia. https//en.wikipedia.org/wiki/Dementia (accessed July 2017).

—. *Silver Alert*. https://en.wikipedia.org/wiki/Silver_Alert (accessed November 29, 2016).

—. *Therapy Dog*. https://en.wikipedia.org/wiki/Therapy_dog (accessed November 29, 2016).

Index

www.ingramcontent.com/pod-product-compliance
Lightning Source LLC
Chambersburg PA
CBHW060840280326
41934CB00007B/866